The
HEALTHY BRAIN
SOLUTION
for
Women Over Forty

The
HEALTHY BRAIN
SOLUTION
for
Women Over Forty

7 Keys to Staying Sharp—
On or Off Hormones

৪০ · ৫৪

Nancy Lonsdorf, MD

Disclaimer

This book provides an educational guide for developing a healthy lifestyle to support healthy brain function. No part of this book is intended to diagnose, prevent or treat any disease or to replace standard medical care. Although preventive in intent, these guidelines do not replace modern preventive medical approaches recommended by your doctor. All information in The Healthy Brain Solution is given with the understanding that the reader accepts full responsibility for her own health and wellbeing. While the self-care approaches outlined in this book have been safely used by hundreds of women, as with any health approach, the results cannot be guaranteed. The author and publisher are not responsible for any adverse effects that may result from food supplements, herbs or dietary and other self-care approaches outlined in this book. Consult with your health-care professional before beginning any herbal products, supplements, remedies, or procedures described in this book and before making any changes in your current medical treatment.

With love and appreciation to all my patients, readers, and course participants—past, present, and future—who keep me inspired with their healthy transformations.

This is for you, in hopes it will guide you, inspire you, and help you create and maintain the healthy brain and sharp cognition you desire and deserve.

Contents

Acknowledgements

The *Healthy Brain Solution for Women Over Forty* comes to meet an urgent need, and I am grateful for the support of all those who came forward to help manifest it quickly. In particular, a big "thank you!" to my patients, staff and family for bearing with me during a time when my attention was focused on writing, and my availability and attention was limited. I am especially appreciative of Patricia Smircich and Maureen Woolley, whose dedicated service, care, and persistence ensured all matters of importance were attended to.

I am thankfully indebted to my editor, Dr. Jocelyne Comtois, for her generous moral support, steadfast encouragement and passionate belief in this book and its purpose. The aid of her extraordinary organizing skills in the face of a vast amount of material, her sharp discrimination, and her support in meeting deadlines were sustaining forces in the forward movement and expeditious completion of this project. A heartfelt thanks to my friend Cynthia Adler, who lent her formidable writing skills on short notice multiples times, sharpening the message, ensuring relevancy, and creating clarity for the lay audience.

I am grateful to Marguerite Plank, who devotedly worked overtime to provide accurate and timely line-editing and for-matting, took edit after edit in stride, and remained cheerfully dedicated to accomplishing the goal. I will always feel deep grat-itude to my magnanimous friend and colleague, Carol Mann, CRNA, for her encouragement and for generously providing an inspiring, nurturing venue with the privacy and quiet I needed to write with full focus on a daily basis. My graphic artist, Margit Trautmann Bown, as always, came through with a beau-tiful and attractive design, and worked dedicatedly to provide quick turnaround on all edits and requests. Randall Zamcheck and Pattie Ptak provided valuable insights regarding supportive online materials and defining the focus of the book.

I thank and acknowledge my many colleagues who are paving the way to a better brain future for everyone. Dr. Dale Bredesen, whose work is revolutionizing Alzheimer's care and will banish this epidemic disease to the historical record, rendering it a rare condition. Dr. Rammohan Rao, whose curiosity and intuitive healing sense led him to study Ayurveda and Alzheimer's, publish the first papers on the topic with Dr. Bredesen, and add Ayurveda's healing power to the cause of reversing cognitive decline. Dr. Mary Kay Ross, who kindly invited my presence in her office and gives generously of her clinical expertise and wisdom. I am grateful to Dr. Sonia Rapaport, whose erudite paper provided a lucid, orderly entree to the complex topic of chronic inflammatory response syndrome and its role in cognitive decline, and who gives freely and open-heartedly of her extensive expertise in this area. Dr. Ann Hathaway shared kindly and liberally of her vast, in-depth knowledge of the role of bioidentical hormones in cognitive health, including their potential value and side-effects. Her diligent adherence to evidence-based decision making and her decidedly science-based presentations drew my attention to the latest evidence, resulting in my growing appreciation of the potential role of bioidenticals in the prevention and treatment of cognitive decline. Thank you, Ann!

My appreciation also goes to: Dr. Robert Keith Wallace, "Dr. Gut," who so clearly articulates the intricacies of the gut-brain connection and fueled my passion for the topic. Dr. Ziv Soferman, who continues to help me discern the emotion-body connection more deeply; to identify the effects of mental and emotional stress on the body, and to understand more fully how to dissolve it. Dr. Fred Travis, whose papers have clarified the many effects of meditation on the brain and especially how different techniques create unique brain benefits.

And finally, my life-long thanks to my mentors in Maharishi Ayurveda over the decades, who have shared selflessly of their deep wisdom, time, clinical expertise, and collegial friendship. I feel truly blessed to have known and worked with the late Dr. Brihaspati Dev Triguna, former President of the All India Ayurveda Congress and personal physician to the President of India and his son, Devendra Triguna, who has followed in his footsteps in both positions and remains dedicated to furthering Ayurveda to help heal the world; Dr. J. R. Raju, whose profound knowledge of pulse diagnosis, and his ability to convey his knowledge fully, via through both styles of teaching—the intuitive Eastern and the logical Western—to Western doctors like myself, gave me a rock-solid foundation in the pulse, for which I'm eternally grateful; the late Dr. Rama Kant Mishra, whose understanding of the sensitivities of the Western physiology, and depth of cognition of the Ayurvedic "workings" of the body, his precisely tuned and highly effective products and his unparalleled ability to teach logically as well as deeply, has been invaluable to my professional development and indispensable to my practice; Dr. Manohar Palakurthi, who is as beloved as he is extraordinary in his understanding of the soul of Ayurveda, the Vedic science underlying Ayurveda, the needs of each patient, and in his highly developed clinical skills and knowledge.

And finally, I acknowledge you, the reader, for stepping up and taking on the challenge of staying sharp throughout your life. And if you have helped me in some special way, I thank you too, and ask your forgiveness for the oversight, as I raise my bottle of Ayurvedic *medhya rasayana* (herbal rejuvenatives for the mind) in salutary salute "to the herbs, the supplements, the ideal diet, the optimal exercise, pure food, water, air, and body, and, most of all, to a happy, healthy brain for us all!"

Foreword

Alzheimer's disease (AD) is a global epidemic affecting nearly 50 million people worldwide. Close to two-thirds of the estimated five million people with Alzheimer's in the U.S are women, and studies indicate that women in their sixties are twice as likely to develop Alzheimer's than to develop breast cancer. While research points to declining estrogen as a causative risk factor for women, there is a lot that is not understood and not yet known.

Meanwhile, more than 5 decades of intensive search for a drug cure has failed to yield any effective treatment for AD. In the past decade alone, hundreds of clinical trials have been conducted, at an aggregate cost of billions of dollars, without success. This has led some to question whether the approach of seeking a drug cure for AD is a viable one. Perhaps a revolutionary new strategy is needed.

The past few decades of genetic and biochemical research have revealed that a multifaceted treatment approach may be a more effective solution to this devastating disease. Data from multiple studies have increasingly pointed to contributors such as insulin resistance, metabolic syndrome, chronic inflammation, vitamin D deficiency, hormone deficiencies and elevated levels of homocysteine. Instead of continuing the futile search for one pill that can somehow modify all the above metabolic contributors, it may be more prudent to embark on a personalized, multitherapy intervention program that addresses each of the modifiable metabolic risk factors.

This book, *The Healthy Brain Solution for Women Over Forty*, provides just such a program.

Dr. Lonsdorf is a Western medical doctor and one of the leading physician advocates of Ayurveda in the United States. She skillfully blends her expertise in Ayurvedic and Western medicine to bring forth the multifaceted approach necessary to provide an effective treatment for this complex disease. The 5,000-year-old science of Ayurveda identifies different physiological and psychological parameters—now shown to be largely genetically based—and prescribes customized lifestyle, diet, and environment most conducive to the well-being of each individual. Combining this knowledge with the latest up-to-date scientific tests and cutting-edge tools available today, this book provides a practical, step-by-step approach to preventing and treating AD.

Using case studies from her own patients, the latest research findings, and Ayurveda, Dr. Lonsdorf provides a holistic, comprehensive, and personalized program consisting of diet, nutritional supplements, spices, yoga, breath practices, sleep, herbs, massage, and the option of bioidentical hormones for healing and empowering the female body, mind, and spirit. The goal of the program is to provide a way for women to lead a simpler, natural, and contented life with a sharp mind and memory, free of Alzheimer's and its impending symptoms.

The successful reversal of cognitive symptoms in patients using this program suggests that an approach of this nature—simple to enact and profound in effect—could be the answer to Alzheimer's many women are seeking. The book not only serves as an authoritative and hopeful guide in our approach to Alzheimer's and its prevention but will also help revolutionize the way we think about and treat this disease.

Rammohan V. Rao, PhD

Alzheimer's researcher and
co-author of scientific papers on Ayurveda and
Alzheimer's Disease with Dale E. Bredesen, MD

Preface

All truth passes through three stages.
First, it is ridiculed.
Second, it is violently opposed.
Third, it is accepted as being self-evident.

—Arthur Schopenhauer

The Healthy Brain Solution for Women Over Forty is designed to empower you with the know-how to prevent, stop, and turn around memory loss in yourself and those you love. You will learn about the first cases of Alzheimer's reversal ever, including regrowth of the memory centers of the brain, and how to apply those same verified healing methods in your life.

The time has arrived when we can prevent, stop, and often even reverse memory loss. Through self-knowledge about our bodies and how to keep them in balance, we can create and live a lifestyle that supports healing.

Alzheimer's first touched my life when I was a young teen. Aunt Barbara, my mom's sister, was visiting, and she, my mom and I were sitting around the kitchen table, enjoying a cup of fresh brew with cardamom coffee cake from the Swedish bakery—a cozy tradition from my grandparents, who had emigrated from "the old country" in the early 1900s.

I knew that Aunt Barbara had recently endured a painful divorce and moved back in with her parents to regroup and raise her four school-aged children as best she could. As if Aunt Barbara didn't have enough with her own challenges, she found herself looking after her aging parents, my beloved Grandma and

Grandpa. After Grandpa died suddenly of a stroke that Christmas, Grandma started to go downhill.

The conversation took a serious turn as Aunt Barbara recounted an incident I will never forget. She related that one day, Grandma was sitting with a caregiver in the living room. As Aunt Barb entered, Grandma glanced up and then turned to her caregiver, fraught with upset and suspicion. "Who is that woman?!" she queried.

"That woman?!" echoed in my mind. Aunt Barbara is her *daughter*, I thought to myself, thoroughly puzzled and disconcerted. How could Grandma possibly not recognize *her own daughter*? I wondered. It sounded, frankly, unbelievable to my 14-year-old ears. It didn't seem plausible, and simply "too cruel" to be true. I pitied my Aunt Barbara and felt sad for Grandma. Perhaps it also struck a deep chord in myself, awakening my young eyes to the tenuousness of our most protective and supportive relationships. I really didn't want the story to be true. Today, thanks to a landmark discovery, it no longer has to be.

Today we are on the brink of an entirely new and refreshing era of self-empowerment regarding our cognitive health. Until now, we've been helpless in the face of memory loss, with no control over our cognitive destiny. Now, a breakthrough discovery is handing us back the reins to our memory—reins that curiously, unbeknownst to us, we have held all along.

Even though we are bombarded by a multitude of headlines declaring the latest touted cause of Alzheimer's—*Is Alzheimer's an Infection? Is Alzheimer's Diabetes of the Brain? Does Air Pollution Cause Alzheimer's?* (all of which may play a role)—yet, to date, no one cause and no one drug has solved the Alzheimer's dilemma. At best, currently available drugs that target one "cause," namely, "grossly low autophagy," deliver temporary improvement, with the disease soon catching up and memory loss resuming, this time with no hope of reprieve.

Which *is* the cause of Alzheimer's? "All of the above" is closer to the truth. Alzheimer's is not one disease, one process, or one cause. It heralds the end result of cumulative assault on our brain cells of over a dozen *different* factors for any one person and the depletion of our enormous "memory reserve" over decades, well before we are even aware that damage is occurring.

Today there is one life-transforming discovery that deserves to capture headlines everywhere (and should be adopted by everyone), that essentially shows that Alzheimer's is an *imbalance* more than a disease. While Alzheimer's as a disease "just happens," memory loss as a physiological *imbalance,* modifiable through diet, supplements, lifestyle—is a revolutionary and empowering insight and has now been validated by published research by Dale Bredesen, MD, of UCLA and the Buck Institute of Aging. This is the *only* approach to date that has documented patients regaining their memory and growing back their brains, in effect, recovering from Alzheimer's.

Today, with women at 100 percent greater risk of Alzheimer's than men, I feel an urgent need to assimilate and share whatever works with my patients, as quickly as possible. This is a disease that does not turn around until *we* act to intercept it. Now we know how, and I've written *The Healthy Brain Solution* to empower you with what you need to know to protect yourself from ever losing your memory, and to recover it if it's waning. The evidence shows it works, and the truth is, the sooner you start, the better the results!

My Path To Reversing Cognitive Decline

As I look back, it has been a long path to this point, both for progress in Alzheimer's research and for my own professional development. For over 30 years, I have been integrating natural approaches, including Ayurveda, the traditional healing system of India and sister science of yoga, into my medical practice.

Natural medicine and Ayurveda have much to offer the unique and oft-neglected health concerns of women, and I've authored and co-authored two books, *A Woman's Best Medicine* and *The Ageless Woman*, to share the healing wisdom of Ayurveda with women of all ages, everywhere.

Moreover, I have always been intrigued by the interplay of mind, body, and health. At my entrance interview to The Johns Hopkins University School of Medicine, at age 19, I shared that I wanted to study what was then the nascent, and somewhat dubious, field of "mind-body medicine," and that I was interested in how the two interact to affect our health and healing. I wanted to go to a school where my interests were supported, and I was willing to risk rejection if it wasn't a match. To my delight, they accepted me despite my avant-garde views. I found Johns Hopkins to be an open-minded, stimulating environment, and received much support for my interests, often far from the mainstream. I elected to specialize in psychiatry, holding "at least they recognize the mind exists." I quickly discovered, however, that I did not want the career I was training for—one dominated by prescribing drugs—so I left the field of psychiatry to study with leading Ayurvedic physicians in India and the U.S., to learn how to heal people in a natural way.

Since then, I have treated over 25,000 patients with Maharishi Ayurveda, the natural health practice from ancient India, along with Western medicine and the added tools of functional medicine (a systematic approach to addressing the root cause of disease, based largely on detailed lab testing of body functioning) to address my patients' needs as fully and holistically as possible.

When I found recently that there was a way to naturally reverse memory loss, I jumped at the opportunity to train with UCLA's Dr. Dale Bredesen, founder of the first truly effective approach to preventing and reversing cognitive decline, and whose natural and holistic approach is in such close alignment with Ayurveda and how I've practiced for over 30 years.

By applying his training in my practice, I quickly began to see positive results. Patients I couldn't help before—and neither could their neurologists—were now getting better! My patients' recoveries have shown me definitively that there is now hope for everyone interested in avoiding Alzheimer's and improving the power of their mind and memory.

To share this breakthrough, I produced a 30-episode live Webinar Intensive called *My Ageless Brain*™, now available as a self-paced, online course. In it, I interview Dr. Bredesen and other experts, as well as guide participants step-by-step through a program informed by the latest evidence-based research. *The Healthy Brain Solution* is here to empower you, and every woman, to avert, stop, and even reverse memory loss.

Very simply, here's how it works...

In this book, you will learn how to discover and eliminate more than 36 identified causes of cognitive decline that you may be vulnerable to. You'll learn the seven essential keys to staying sharp after 40, including how to heal your gut, optimize your blood sugar, squelch inflammation, replenish vital nutrients and hormones, and eliminate toxins. You will learn the latest about the risks and benefits of bioidentical hormones—when best to start, if at all, and when to stop, if appropriate.

Each chapter ends with a short "one-minute summary," and a link to online resources to complement your healing journey. With proven strategies and directions guiding you step by step, you'll tip your brain's inner balance towards building brain cells and memory power, while you boost your overall health and vitality. If you are concerned about memory loss, have a family history of Alzheimer's, or simply want to sharpen your memory, feel great, and look younger than you really are, this book is for you.

1

Memory Loss Is Preventable

No one loses memory for no reason.

—Dale Bredesen, MD

Key #1: Identify and Remedy Your Risks

There is good news on the horizon for women's health. A new therapeutic breakthrough stands to eliminate one of the most heart-breaking diseases, one that currently takes the lives of one in seven American women over 65. For the first time in the long history of this relentless disease, despite billions spent on failed drug trials, a treatment modality has finally been identified that can actually stop and even reverse Alzheimer's previously inexorable decline.

And the "cure" is *not* the usual high-tech medical break-through of expensive drugs, immune therapy, or gene therapy, as we may think. Rather, the solution is an amazingly low tech, multimodality, natural approach that is within the reach of you, me, and everyone right now.

Pioneering "Patient Zero"—Kristin's Story

Under the soft southern California sky, Eliza Bruner related the dramatic story of her best friend, Kristin (not their real names). In short, Kristin was a 68-year-old globetrotting, high-level consultant who spoke seven languages, and had a very successful professional career. Yet, Kristin called Eliza one day in a panic—she had taken a flight cross-country, arrived at the airport, and couldn't remember why she was there or who she was there to see. Unable to figure it out, she caught the next flight back to her home on the East Coast. Only when she reviewed her messages at home did she realize with whom she was supposed to meet and why. Kristin's eventual diagnosis was not good. She had Alzheimer's disease.

Devastated, Kristin remembered her mother's long, protracted suffering and eventual death from Alzheimer's, that she herself had nurtured her through. She did not want to put her family through that, and she could not accept it for herself, so she called Eliza to say good-bye. She was going to take her own life.

"Wait a minute," Eliza pleaded, I know someone who might be able to help you. She told Kristin about Dr. Bredesen's multimodal, lifestyle-based research protocol, as yet untested because no drug company would fund a study. As a result of Eliza's urgent plea, Dr. Bredesen agreed to try his multimodal protocol for the very first time, with Kristin as the one and only subject. They met and talked for several hours. At the end, Dr. Bredesen gave Kristin a comprehensive profile of blood tests to do—to check for underlying inflammation, blood sugar issues, deficiencies, and toxic exposure—and a behavioral prescription that included restarting her lapsed hormone therapy, regular exercise, a whole-food diet, multiple supplements, and re-establishing her regular practice of Transcendental Meditation.

Amazingly, within a few months, Kristin reported that her memory was recovering. She could keep her pets' names straight, hold numbers in her head again, and remember her grocery list. Soon, she was again able to understand complex reports at work. She began yoga and enrolled in a yoga therapist training program, which she successfully completed. She eventually regained all of her cognitive abilities and returned to intellectually challenging, full-time work, teaching at a major university at the age of 75.

I was stunned by Kristin's story. As a physician, I assumed that Alzheimer's was incurable. Hearing Kristin's touching and dramatic story of recovery filled me with hope and possibility. With my tools of Ayurveda, functional medicine, mind-body coaching, and Transcendental Meditation, I had helped many thousands of patients with chronic diseases who otherwise were not getting better. Now I realized that the incurable Alzheimer's disease could be reversed *with the very tools and approaches I use every day in my practice.* Here was hope indeed.

Nevertheless, as a doctor, I knew that Kristin's recovery was just a story, a case report. I would need more evidence, and training, to go further. I filed Kristin's remarkable story away and went back to my practice. I had no thought that soon I, too, would be seeing such "miraculous" turnarounds in my patients with cognitive decline.

Yet, a few months later, I got wind that Dr. Bredesen himself was teaching doctors his protocol at The Institute for Functional Medicine's *Advanced Clinical Training in Reversing Cognitive Decline* in Dallas, Texas. I was thrilled! I immediately booked a flight and spent two fascinating days with Dr. Bredesen and his colleagues, learning how to turn around Alzheimer's disease. I feel fortunate to have studied firsthand with the scientist who had the breakthrough insight that Alzheimer's would never be cured with a single drug. Since Alzheimer's disease results from *dozens* of causes, not just one mechanism, one "active ingredient" can never fix it.

I was excited to bring this new powerful skill set back to my practice. I hoped I would see the kinds of results Dr. Bredesen presented, in my own patients. While I had helped reverse memory loss in a handful who had heavy metal toxicity, B12 deficiency, or were taking memory-damaging medications, I needed a reliable protocol that could help nearly anyone. That protocol had finally arrived.

The Discovery—Alzheimer's Can Be Reversed

Dr. Dale Bredesen evolved his multimodality approach of diet, supplements, and lifestyle changes through working with Kristin and the dozens who followed her.

He published his first case series in 2014 in the prestigious *Journal of Aging,* in which he documented reversal of cognitive decline in 9 of 10 patients. In 2016, he published another case series, including MRI findings that demonstrated the remarkable fact that the brain can grow back its memory center—the hippocampus—an astounding discovery. One patient improved from a starting hippocampal volume of only the 17th percentile for his age to a repeat scan only 10 months later in the 75th percentile—a remarkable achievement indeed!

Since then, Dr. Bredesen and clinical colleagues have treated over 200 patients using his multimodal approach, customizing treatment via extensive blood tests that help identify the unique combination of potential contributors present for each individual.

In 2018, Dr. Bredesen and colleagues published yet another paper, "Reversal of Cognitive Decline: 100 patients," in the *Journal of Alzheimer's Disease and Parkinsonism,* further documenting improvements in over 100 additional patients using his protocol. In 2018, Dr. Bredesen published his latest research in the *Journal of Alzheimer's Disease and Parkinsonism.* The paper, "Reversal of Cognitive Decline: 100 patients," documents functional improvements in 100 patients diagnosed with varying levels of cognitive decline, and further supports the effectiveness of the protocol used in the treatment of all patients involved in the study.

The Healthy Brain Solution is based on Dr. Bredesen's integrative, multimodality program, as taught by him and his colleagues at The Institute for Functional Medicine, plus the Ayurvedic wisdom I have found to be transformational to the health of my patients over the past three decades.

This book provides a revolutionary, highly doable program to slow and even reverse Alzheimer's usual relentless, progressive course. By identifying your vulnerabilities, and correcting them now, you no longer have to fear or face a future of memory loss and cognitive decline.

How Can Alzheimer's Possibly Be Reversed Without a Miracle Drug?

How can supplements and lifestyle changes possibly solve an "incurable" condition, you may wonder. Steeped in our culture of "magic bullet" drug treatments, such an approach may sound implausible, yet it's leading to real results in real patients. Let's consider how it can work.

We are accustomed to thinking about disease in terms of a single molecule or mechanism. Autoimmune disease, prevalent dogma holds, is due to the body somehow "attacking itself" with self-directed antibodies. The *immune system* itself is labeled as the problem and potent drugs are given to suppress it. Heart disease is due to cholesterol, that *villainous* molecule that clogs our arteries and creates heart attacks and strokes. We are given drugs to block its production.

In the case of Alzheimer's disease, another "rogue" molecule takes the brunt of the blame, sticky amyloid-beta (or, for simplicity's sake, "amyloid"), builds up between neurons in the brain, causing them to shrivel up and die. Yet, counterintuitively, simply removing the amyloid with drugs hasn't helped, and in some cases, even worsens the disease.

Let's challenge this "villain" model of disease. Our immune system can hardly be held culpable for purposely harming us; indeed, its very purpose is to protect us. *Bad* immune system? Indeed, recent research on the classic autoimmune disease *rheumatoid arthritis* is toppling the idea of a "confused" immune system with evidence that the gut microbiome and intricately related mechanisms play an important role in— and may even trigger—the disease.

Likewise, cholesterol itself is hardly an enemy we have to get rid of. A full 25 percent of the body's cholesterol is located in the brain, which comprises a mere 3 percent of our body weight. Cholesterol is a key component that coats and protects our cell membranes, including neurons, and is the primary building block of our steroid hormones. We need cholesterol, and plenty of it, to make our estrogen, progesterone, testosterone, cortisol, and vitamin D. Cholesterol is anything but a "bad guy." *We cannot live without cholesterol* and some patients report that lowering it too much adversely affects their cognition, sleep, or mood. It is not that our miraculous human body is fundamentally flawed and prone to irreversible disease. Rather, it's our way of thinking about disease, our *model* of disease that's falling short.

Disease doesn't "just happen." We are designed to be healthy and stay healthy, and will, as long as we give our bodies the proper nourishment, sleep, balanced activity, love, and social interaction they thrive on. Disease is nearly always a result of preventable factors, not an inevitability. To correct it, we have to remove the causes and activate the body's own healing mechanisms to reverse the processes that deteriorated it in the first place. And, remarkably, in most cases, if it's not too far advanced, the body (and brain) can bounce back!

Doesn't Amyloid Cause Alzheimer's?

In the case of Alzheimer's disease, it is not as simple as pointing the finger at amyloid as the problem and attacking, removing, or inhibiting its deposition with a drug. If it were, plenty of anti-amyloid drugs would have cured it by now.

In the early 2000s, Robert Moir and Rudolf Tanzi of Harvard Medical School had the sudden insight that the body's innate immune system may be involved in Alzheimer's disease. In fact, when they looked into it further, they found that a key molecule of the innate immune system had a structure almost identical to amyloid, and further study showed that *without* amyloid, animals exposed to certain brain infections would die, whereas those *with* amyloid survived.

The revolutionary idea that amyloid itself is an integral part of our brain's inborn immune response has been recognized as the brainchild of these two brilliant, independent-minded scientists. In a landmark paper with Soscia et al., they demonstrate that amyloid is a powerful antimicrobial that serves to protect the brain from viruses and bacteria. Could it be that amyloid is actually something innately *good* and Alzheimer's represents a fundamentally *protective* mechanism gone out of hand?

That is exactly the viewpoint of Dr. Dale Bredesen, who attributes Alzheimer's disease to a condition of "balance lost" in an otherwise healthy physiological process, not unlike what happens in osteoporosis. Normal bone systematically breaks down "old bone" and replaces it with fresh, stronger "new" bone in a balanced fashion that maintains normal bone mass. In osteoporosis, however, the normal balance tips in the direction of breakdown, leading to progressive thinning of the bones over time.

In the case of Alzheimer's, amyloid becomes problematic only when the body makes too much of it. Excess amyloid clumps together, clogging the spaces between neurons and sending out too many signals to the brain to "downsize." Whereas a healthy brain keeps itself in balance via two contrasting critical processes: building new connections (creating memories and learning) and breaking down connections (forgetting irrelevant details), in Alzheimer's, the breaking down of connections *exceeds* the building up. The initial result is loss of the ability to learn new things and remember them. Then, progressively, more and more important memories, learned skills, and abilities disappear.

7

This idea of innate balance, and evidence supporting it, is highly fulfilling to my "Ayurvedic ears" as Ayurvedic theory is founded on the concept of *balance* as the basis of health. Furthermore, one of my most influential teachers, Dr. J. R. Raju, taught in a special Ayurvedic pulse course for doctors these important instructions: When evaluating a patient, we must always keep in mind that we are not only seeing the disease, and the patient with the disease, but also the body's attempt to heal itself, including the body's response to what is attempting to drive it out of balance—the body's attempts to heal itself. For example, fever, purulence, rashes, and so on, are all signs of the body's immune system at work against an invader. He emphasized how important it was that we keep in mind this principle in all our patient work, "The body is *always* trying to heal itself."

So here, thousands of years after Ayurvedic knowledge was first conceived, a fundamental Ayurvedic tenet is helping illuminate the path to one of the most enigmatic and elusive "cures" of all time. The unique dimension of healing that is Ayurveda is as relevant to our healing today as it was 5,000 years ago.

Now, let's look further into what drives the body's protective immune process that results in *too much* amyloid, and what it means for our health. I think you'll find it extremely empowering to know that *we* ourselves stand at the helm of the forces that drive our brain's amyloid production. If we are making too much, it is now possible to identify why and to correct the problem at its source.

Here's how it works …

It's All About *Balance*

The story begins with a *pre*-amyloid molecule called "amyloid precursor protein," or APP for short. APP is a receptor, meaning, like a lock, it "receives" various molecules that fit into it, like a key. More than one type of "key" can activate the

APP receptor, and depending on which "key" inserts itself, APP responds by breaking into either an amyloid-forming option or a nerve-growing option—very different outcomes, indeed. APP is found on every cell membrane of the brain, especially near synapses, where neurons connect. The role of APP is decisive. Its "breaking" determines whether the cells around it grow and connect or retract and cower for protection, eventually to die if the intended milieu does not become more favorable.

If the brain is flooded predominantly with wholesome nutrients, replete with hormones and other nourishment it needs to thrive, then APP will be broken down into just *two pieces*. This "dynamic duo" promotes neuronal growth and connection, enabling us to learn and remember new things.

Alternatively, challenge it with an onslaught of threatening viruses, bacteria, heavy metals or other toxins, and APP will instead be cleaved into a "quarreling quartet" of four tiny by-products, *including amyloid* itself. Amyloid, and its fellow quartet members, signal surrounding neurons to "retract and protect," similar to a tortoise that pulls his head into his shell when threatened. To add insult to injury, newly formed amyloid *bites back* on surrounding APP molecules, triggering *them* to break into "quarreling quartets," which in turn beget more amyloid. It's a vicious cycle that we can, and *must*, dismantle by giving the body the highest value in our daily food and lifestyle choices, as well as targeted supplements, nutrients, and hormones, according to each person's unique needs as we age.

In summary, whether our brain makes neuron-destroying amyloid or "memory-making molecules" depends on our inner brain milieu. The good news is, that inner environment depends a lot on *us*. How we eat, sleep, and live results in real, immediate impact—either up or down—on amyloid production in our brains.

When we eat and live healthfully, we support whole-brain and whole-body health, strengthening the mind, memory, and *growth-promoting* brain chemistry such as growth hormone, and melatonin. On the other hand, if we consume unwholesome foods, short our sleep, slack on exercise, and breathe polluted air, for just example, we will likely push our APP in the direction of more and more amyloid.

Amyloid: Protect us it will. Immune function it has. Sticky, cloggy, and destructive (in excess) it is. Amyloid is all of this. The key here is *balance.* To keep amyloid in our favor, we need to keep our lives in balance. Too much amyloid simply means there are too many toxic or infectious influences assaulting your brain and too few vital nutrients and hormones to nourish, clean, and protect it.

My First "Patient Zero"—Catherine's Story

Soon after I began my Bredesen program practice, Catherine, an 80-year-old retired yoga teacher, came to see me in despair, at the urging of her children. "They're concerned that I'm not following their conversations, that I'm not getting what they want to get across to me."

Earlier that year, Catherine had undergone life-saving open-heart surgery for a double bypass and a valve replacement. She confessed that she now felt so weak and "not herself" that sometimes she wondered if she should have done it at all.

She went on to relate, "I don't go out anymore. I was going to the local natural food store, and a few times I ran into people that I knew, or I thought I knew. I would say hi to them by name, but they weren't the person I thought they were. It was very embarrassing. I just stopped going."

She also described difficulty with directions and spatial orientation. When in the basement, for example, she had trouble figuring out where the other floors of her house were.

Her MoCA score (Montreal Cognitive Assessment, a simple verbal, paper-and-pencil test I gave her in the office) was 25, consistent with mild cognitive impairment.

Catherine had read about the new scientific evidence that memory problems could be reversed. She came ready to do everything she needed to get better, even on her limited budget. In the first visit, Catherine got orders for comprehensive blood tests to assess for inflammation, blood sugar control, nutrient and hormone levels, and heavy metals. (See the following sidebar, "My Online Resources for You.")

My Online Resources for You: "The Cognoscopy" lab tests

Go to www.thehealthybrainsolution.com for a free, downloadable and printable PDF that lists the comprehensive lab tests I typically order for my patients. You can bring a copy to your doctor or use it yourself as a guide to ordering self-test kits online.

At the site, you'll also get the "Basic Lab Test List" that itemizes those tests I consider the *minimum essential starting point*—budget-friendly and often covered by insurance. Your doctor may be willing to order these tests for you, as they are in line with "standard" tests he or she is used to ordering. In order to be covered by your insurance, your doctor will need to provide a diagnosis code that matches the criterion your insurance company sets for each test.

Diagnosis codes, however, are selected according to the medical conditions and symptoms you have, so don't always meet the lab's requirements. The lab can usually tell you at the time you go for your blood draw, which tests insurance will not cover, based on the diagnosis codes your doctor provided. If you are on Medicare, they must by law inform you of the tests that are not likely to be covered and get your permission and payment commitment if you decide to go ahead with the test anyway.

Note re: "Optimal Test Levels"—These lab test lists also contain *optimal* lab values for each test, meaning the levels you need for optimal brain benefit—not simply the accepted "norm" for the population, as provided by the lab.

We also discussed highly personalized dietary, herbal, and behavioral steps, and individualized Ayurvedic supplements that she could take right away. She especially liked the idea of getting back to regular *pranayama,* a yoga breathing technique she had gotten away from. She mentioned that a master yoga instructor of hers once had recommended pranayama for another student's mother, who had memory problems, and she intuitively felt it would be good for her.

After her test results returned, she began supplements to correct low adrenal hormones, iron deficiency anemia, border-line low B12 and other B vitamins, and a low-grade urinary tract infection. Her lead level was borderline high, so I recommended a program of supplements to help her body gently, but effec-tively, eliminate that.

Just two weeks later, something remarkable and very mean-ingful happened to her. She was doing her chosen "brain train-ing," which was studying Sanskrit chants, some of which she had learned many years ago. She hadn't been able to remember any "by heart" for years, and not for want of trying. She had a favorite that she really wanted to recall, but "for the life of me, I couldn't." Then, all of a sudden, out of nowhere, "it came back to me. And not just parts of it, the whole thing."

Catherine was, needless to say, extremely delighted with this and even sang the chant for me on video. When Catherine told me this experience, I got goosebumps. It was almost word-for-word the experience of a young woman Dr. Bredesen had introduced during our training—a lady who had experienced facial recognition problems as Catherine did, and had wanted to remember the Russian she learned in college but couldn't recall even a word. Then one day, all of a sudden, her Russian "came back. And not just part of it, all of it."

Another two months later, Catherine reported that she was doing 30 minutes of pranayama twice a day, taking all her sup-plements as prescribed, and practicing her Transcendental Medi-tation twice a day, after pranayama. She even started to do a few yoga poses again.

In conclusion, she wrote, "As a result of the program, my mind is noticeably clearer and stronger. Chants I used to know and love suddenly came back to me. I now recognize friends I see in public. I enjoy people more, and I am more talkative and more fluent in my conversations with people. I still have some 'blanks,' but I'm confident those will get better, too. I am very happy I started this program!"

The Three (and One-Half) Subtypes of Alzheimer's Disease

In Dr. Bredesen's nearly 30 years of basic science research on Alzheimer's disease, he discovered no fewer than 36 factors that can drive the production of amyloid. Like "36 holes in a roof," he described that correcting one, two, or three of these causative factors with a drug (the best a drug can be expected to do), is like patching only three of the 36 holes in the roof and expecting no water to leak through anymore.

Rather, Dr. Bredesen developed his multifaceted approach specifically to "patch" all the holes and proposed *three main disease processes* that increase amyloid production and eventually lead to Alzheimer's disease.

According to Bredesen, Alzheimer's disease can be broken down into three main subtypes, based on the cause (inflammatory, atrophic, and toxic) or six subtypes, if including glycotoxic, vascular, and traumatic. Identifying your predominant subtypes can help you and your doctor develop an individualized treatment approach to prevent or reverse the symptoms associated with each.

Doing the comprehensive profile of tests, the "cognoscopy" (see "Month One, Key #1" in Chapter Eight), will give you the information you need to identify and correct your vulnerabilities. Most people have hormonal imbalances, deficiencies, influences, or other impacts that span across a number of subtypes. If you can't identify your subtype, no worries! It is more important to do your tests and optimize your values with the help of your doctor.

For a summary of distinguishing features of each type, refer to Table 1. Meanwhile, let's consider what you need to do next.

Table 1. Subtypes of Alzheimer's Disease	
Type 1:	Inflammatory ("Hot"). It occurs more often in people who carry one or two ApoE4 alleles and tends to run in families. This type typically begins with a loss of the ability to store new information. Symptoms often begin in the late forties or fifties.
Type 2:	Atrophic ("Cold"). Loss of ability to form new memories appears about a decade later than the inflammatory type. There is no inflammation but the overall support for brain synapses has dried up. Hormone levels are low, vitamin D is reduced, insulin resistance may occur, and insulin level is low. Homocysteine associated with brain atrophy and Alzheimer's disease may be high.
Type 1.5:	Glycotoxic ("Sweet"). Combines features and causes of Types 1 and 2. ApoE4 is an important risk factor. Patients have poor short-term memory, learning, and orientation. Inflammation is present and there are problems with insulin resistance. When insulin resistant, not only does the body handle sugar poorly, but brain cells lose an important "trophic factor," as insulin otherwise acts to support their growth. One of the most common contributors to cognitive decline today is insulin resistance.
Type 3:	Toxic ("Vile"). This subtype tends to occur in those at average risk genetically, with both copies of ApoE3/3. This type does not run in families. Type 3 usually begins in the late 40s to early 60s, often precipitated by excessive stress and exposure to toxins (mercury, mycotoxins, Lyme, surgical implants, chronic viral infections). Patients lose recent and old memories and how to do complex things, even simple ones like speaking. Depression, trouble focusing, worsening when under stress, and attention deficit are also common.

Type 4:	Vascular ("Pale"). Heart disease and stroke appear to hasten the risk of cognitive decline in normal older individuals. Early symptoms are typically not isolated to short-term memory and can be diverse such as difficulty following directions, doing familiar tasks, losing orientation while driving, uncontrolled laughing or crying, impaired planning and judgement, speech difficulties, etc.
Type 5:	Traumatic ("Dazed"). Research has linked multiple, moderate, or severe traumatic brain injury to a greater risk of developing Alzheimer's or another type of dementia years after the original head injury.

What Should You Do Next?

Once you identify your risk factors and insulin vulnerabilities and correct them, you have effectively "cut the disease off at the root." Rather than simply spraying "leaf polish" on the surface of the problem, as drugs do today, you are addressing and eliminating the real underlying causes—and what better prevention can there be?

How should you go about "immunizing" yourself from Alzheimer's disease? Clearly, we want to begin to live the principle in our daily lives of "in with the good, out with the bad."

In general, adopting a whole-foods, organic, plant-based diet, good sleep habits, regular exercise, brain training, and effectively managing stress are all critical for your neurons to grow and thrive. If your nutrients or hormones are found to be too low, you will need to consult your doctor about safely correcting these deficiencies.

Likewise, eliminating "bad" fats, unhealthy oils, and deep-fried foods, environmental chemicals, mold, and hidden infections, along with correcting your nutritional and hormonal deficiencies, and countering excess stress, will help prevent your brain from "downsizing" and clogging up with memory-busting amyloid protein.

Why Start So Early As Age 40...?

This book is specifically for women over 40. Why start as young as 40? For a problem so far in the future, most of us would prefer to forget about it for another 20 years. Simply put, we cannot afford to wait. A growing body of research indicates that deterioration of the brain starts as long as 20 years before memory loss sets in—long before you know anything is wrong.

Our ever-changing hormonal milieu may put us at increased risk—women now get Alzheimer's at twice the rate of men. Menopause has a major impact on our hormones, and even in the decades that follow, levels continue to slowly, gradually decline. Recent research has documented an alarming deterioration in memory regions of the brain in normal women approaching and passing through menopause, while their age-matched male peers did *not* undergo such accelerated decline. We'll discuss specific ways to support balance and counter decline during this peri-menopausal time in Chapter Six.

If 40 is not too early, could 80 be too late? While Bredesen's research indicates chances of a turnaround are greatest before age 75, Catherine, at age 80, was fortunate to be able to turn her cognitive symptoms around, and quickly. Perhaps it was her many years of yoga practice, Transcendental Meditation, and wholesome organic diet, or her personal determination to "do whatever it takes" and follow the regimen fully. I have found that those who adopt the program "full out" get the best results, just as Catherine did.

Generally speaking, this program works best for those under 75 years old and in the early stages of cognitive decline. That includes both those with MCI, mild cognitive impairment (when tests show impaired cognition, but the person lives her life more or less normally) or early Alzheimer's (when the person is impaired to the point that she is no longer fully able to perform her daily activities independently, but can lead a fairly normal life with assistance).

Now we know that cognitive decline is not caused by just one "elusive" factor, but usually a dozen or more, all simultaneously triggering more and more amyloid production in the brain's attempts to protect itself. It's an *additive* and cumulative process that we can "head off at the pass" early on by identifying what may be causing it for ourselves, even if we don't have—and may never get—dementia down the line. Correcting your factors *now* carries the side benefits of a sharper mind, better focus, more energy and vitality, and an all-around healthier YOU.

More Specifically, I Recommend That You...

First, I highly encourage you identify any underlying deficiencies or potential causes of current or future cognitive decline by undergoing thorough testing (mainly blood tests you can do through your local doctor). You can also order kits online, without need for your doctor's order (but also not usually coverable by insurance) that you can take to your local hospital or designated lab service center. They will draw and process your blood and then report the results, which you can share with your health care practitioner.

Once you know what nutrients or hormones you may be deficient in, and whether you have excess inflammation, a newly discovered chronic infection, or other abnormality, see your doctor for personalized guidance. At the same time, make sure you check out upcoming chapters that may be relevant to your situation. Write down the questions you want to ask your doctor and be your own best advocate.

If you're low in brain-critical nutrients or have hormonal deficiencies, your own doctor may feel comfortable prescribing fortifying supplements or bioidentical replacement hormones (there are bioidentical options available through standard pharmacies today.) If not, you may want to seek out a doctor trained in bioidentical hormone therapy, which we'll talk more about in Chapter Six.

If there's evidence of heavy metal toxicity, mold exposure or other biotoxicity, you may wish to see a functional medicine specialist to guide you through the complexities of clearing it out and restoring optimal health.

In Summary...

This book is laid out to take you step by step through the potential causes of Alzheimer's and cognitive decline, including the specific tests that will assess your risk with regard to each potential cause. Relevant tests and action steps are summarized in Chapter Eight, with a suggested "7-Month" plan that mirrors the first seven chapters in this book, providing all seven keys you need to stay sharp after 40—yes—*on or off* hormones. Flip back to Chapter Eight whenever you wish to order a test for yourself or for a quick summary of what you need to get one of the seven keys "covered."

Once your test results return, you'll want to correct any identified vulnerabilities with personalized diet, lifestyle, supplements, and other therapies as needed. As always, be sure to check with your doctor before beginning a new supplement, diet or exercise program, particularly if you have a medical condition or take medication.

Keep in mind that benefits have not only been subjective but objectively verified. Published research has documented that atrophied brain areas, such as the hippocampus, a vital memory center, have actually *grown back* as a result of diet, targeted supplements, and lifestyle, including stress-reduction.

Is Testing Beyond Your Budget Right Now? *Or* Are You "Test Phobic?"

No worries! While I highly recommend, as I've done myself, undergoing the full panel of tests that Dr. Bredesen playfully dubbed the "cognoscopy" (a term I will use to denote the comprehensive testing outlined in this book), if for some reason you do not do the whole panel at this time, you will still get tremendous value from becoming conversant with the main underlying causes of cognitive decline and adopting the diet and lifestyle measures outlined here to prevent them.

This book is designed for you to proceed chapter by chapter, systematically addressing each potential contributor to cognitive decline. You'll learn what tests to do—if you want to—and what steps you should take in order to protect yourself from the potentially damaging effects of that particular cause over time. You will, in effect, be "immunizing" yourself—according to the best knowledge we have today—against future cognitive decline. At the same time, you'll be creating optimal health for yourself and your precious brain, making it possible to enjoy your life, even more, today!

Take This Simple Action #1 Now!

Go to *www.thehealthybrainsolution.com* and download your free, printable PDF of the Comprehensive Lab Tests I typically order for Healthy Brain preventive evaluation.

You can bring a copy to your doctor or use it as a guide to ordering "self-test" kits online. Here's one easy step that will set you on the path of healthy, sharp mind, brain and memory for a lifetime.

www.thehealthybrainsolution.com

Like a video about this breakthrough discovery?
Tune into *My Ageless Brain* master class at
https://myagelessbrain.com/free-masterclass/

2

Inflammation and Your Brain

Without proper diet, medicines are of no use.
With proper diet, medicines are of no need.

—Ayurvedic aphorism

Key #2: Balance Your Inflammatory Response

Our bodies are self-healing systems by design. Scrape your skin and it reddens, heralding new skin soon to appear. Bruise your shin and it swells before the bruise fades and disappears. Get a virus and your body expels it with an intricate defense of fever, mucus, coughs, and sneezes.

As a species, we humans have survived innumerable assaults from injury, infection, and climate change. Today we face perhaps our most insidious threat yet, progressive deterioration from chronic disease, largely "lifestyle disease" of our own making.

The protective, life-saving immune response that has healed us from time immemorial now threatens to destroy our bodies, our brains, and our minds. Overstimulated by modern living and an unprecedented onslaught of environmental toxins, our immune systems are all too likely to *over-do* the lofty protective role they were designed for. The result in our brains, bodies, arteries, and gut is a "fire" burning out of control—*inflammation on overdrive.*

21

Inflammation—or overactivity of the immune system—is implicated as one of the most important drivers today of cognitive decline, brain deterioration, and Alzheimer's disease.

As women at risk, we must protect our brains proactively, by adopting an "anti-inflammatory" diet and lifestyle. (You'll get tips and strategies later in this chapter.) It is also helpful, and can be very motivating, to objectively measure the level of inflammation in your body right now, through appropriate blood tests, as listed at the end of this chapter. If elevated, no worries! Adjusting your diet, lifestyle, and taking supplements, if needed, can help squelch the "flames" and get your immune response back in balance.

Before we further address practical steps, let's understand more deeply what inflammation *is* and how and why we must keep it in balance.

Nature Didn't Make "Bad"

Inflammation serves us every day. Whatever the challenge, our bodies respond with one common pathway—inflammation. It is our body's own protective response—our healing system at work. Inflammation is our body's shock troops—our "good guys" striving to defeat any invader set upon doing our bodies harm. As with an indomitable national defense, inflammation must render us impenetrable to the enemy. Our lives depend on it.

Yet inflammation has *un*deservedly become the new villain in disease theory. "Undeservedly," because inflammation in and of itself is not bad—nor is it good. It's simply necessary to life. But ... for ideal health, it *must* be kept in balance.

While we need inflammation for occasional assaults on the body from sudden injury, stress, infection, or toxic exposure, it is *not* meant to be activated on a daily basis. Poor diet, mental stress, overwork, lack of sleep and exercise, excess alcohol, and recreational chemicals are a few all-too-common features of our everyday lifestyle that contribute to chronic inflammation.

We need a healthy, strong, vital, *but* not overly reactive immune system. Too much inflammation produces "friendly fire" that can damage our own body tissues, not just the unwelcome invader.

When modern lifestyle leads to chronic inflammation, "friendly fire" from an overzealous immune response can affect nearly any area of the body. Chronic inflammation can result in such diverse conditions as arthritis, asthma, allergies, eczema, colitis, endometriosis, heart disease, and cancer. Lately, scientific research has linked inflammation to brain-related conditions such as depression and neurodegenerative diseases, including Alzheimer's and Parkinson's disease. The many ways our brain is affected by inflammation is becoming clearer as scientific research progresses.

Your Brain *On Fire*

Inflammation in the brain is increasingly regarded as an essential ingredient for amyloid deposition in Alzheimer's, and many risk factors are known to trigger it, not the least of which is the food we eat and the lifestyles we lead. In fact, evidence points to inflammation as both a cause and result of amyloid deposition, as amyloid itself stimulates more inflammation in a vicious cycle akin to *"adding gasoline to a fire."*

Researchers Wyss-Coray and Rogers, in their *Brief Review* of published studies on inflammation and Alzheimer's disease (AD), found that nearly one-third of over 20,000 total studies on Alzheimer's were dedicated to inflammation. "If nothing else, the burgeoning number of papers on inflammation and AD that are summarized in this review make plain the remarkable complexity of inflammatory mechanisms in AD and the many challenges that such complexity imposes with respect to selecting or developing appropriate therapeutics."

It's worth pointing out again that 20,000 research papers, billions of dollars, and decades of brilliant minds working around the clock have thus far failed to uncover the one "magic bullet" that can cure AD, stop its progression, or even prevent it.

With our knowledge today, however, that inflammation plays a major role in our brain health, as do blood sugar, hormones, nutrients, and toxins, we don't have to wait for scientists, government officials, funding organizations, or insurance companies to "sign off" on a multi-cause model of Alzheimer's disease, or to fund a multimodal approach to preventing and reversing it, (though it will be helpful when they do!)

Rather, the time to take charge of our brain health is *now*. We are in the driver's seat—cognitive vitality is within our grasp. We already *know* how to reduce inflammation—food, air, exercise, stress, body fat and sleep all powerfully influence our bodies' inflammatory response. Fortunately, we are no longer helpless in the face of the enemy. *We* are more powerful than we ever imagined, more powerful than any pill ever will be.

How Inflammation Can Cause "Brain Fog": An Example

When the immune system is in overdrive in one part of the body, distant brain effects may also be present that had not been fully appreciated in the past. Let's consider, for example, rheumatoid arthritis, a chronic autoimmune, inflammatory condition that is commonly considered a joint disease. To investigate how systemic inflammation may affect the brain, researchers at Michigan Medicine's Chronic Pain and Fatigue Research Center compared brain scans of subjects with rheumatoid arthritis to levels of inflammation in the peripheral blood.

Of 264 brain regions studied, inflammation was found to mostly affect the inferior parietal lobe and the medial prefrontal cortex, areas associated with what patients called "brain fog." These areas are involved in visuospatial processing, decision making, and memory retrieval. The researchers concluded that inflammation as measured in the peripheral blood tests may be altering functional connections in the brain, interfering with mental clarity.

Research has found that consumption of a healthy Mediterranean-like diet high in plant-based foods, healthy fats, and spices led to a significant improvement in immune function. It has also shown that exercise and healthy sleeping habits, as well as stress reduction modalities, work to reduce stress hormones and support a healthy, balanced immune response. The consequent benefits to mental clarity can be very quick and direct.

Jeannie's Story—Simple, Elegant, Amazingly Fast

Jeannie is a 68-year-old social worker and mother of five who joined my one-on-one Healthy Brain Program to turn around a decline in her memory she had been noticing over the previous year. She was very concerned about it because her mother had died of Alzheimer's. At the end of her life, she could not even recognize family members, a very frightening and depressing thought to Jeannie, to whom family meant everything. Jeannie herself tells her story:

> I had been noticing that numbers had become really very difficult for me. I would be working on the computer and look at a 4- to 6-digit number and think I would transfer it to another place in the computer. By the time I got over there, I couldn't remember it. I was also having trouble with words. As I was talking and giving speeches, and leading in-service trainings, I noticed that I couldn't think of the word I needed and then would have to engage the audience to have them help me say what I wanted to say.
>
> I was also having trouble with remembering. I would be sitting somewhere, and I would think, "I have to remember

this. I want to add this to my list," because I'm a list person. By the time I got to paper and pen, I had forgotten what I was going to put on that list.

Timelines were difficult, trying to remember what had happened in the last week, the last month, the last several months. Short-term memory was very difficult for me. I found myself re-reading books that I had read two or three months before. Then my daughter would say, "Well, we just read that book. Don't you remember?" I'd say, "Oh, I vaguely remember that." So I was losing a lot of those kind of thought processes, and that concerned me.

After evaluating Jeannie in her first visit, I gave her orders for a comprehensive set of blood tests, the "cognoscopy." I also encouraged her to continue her long-time practice of Transcendental Meditation for deep relaxation, and gave her initial, customized recommendations based on her Ayurvedic evaluation—her mind-body type and the imbalances evident through *pulse assessment,* a traditional technique that allows a glimpse into the physiology, even before detailed bloodwork returns.

From her pulse, I could immediately see that Jeannie had considerable inflammation in her body, and a "clogginess" Ayurveda terms *ama.* Ama is defined as "undigested food," food that was not completely broken down into the finest particles of fatty acids, amino acids, and sugars before it was absorbed.

Ama can enter the circulation inappropriately through the gut wall, lodge in tissues such as joints and sinuses, and cause inflammation and disease. Remarkably similar to our current understanding of "leaky gut," Ayurveda knew it all thousands of years ago.

Jeannie had "earned" her ama through poor eating habits since moving in with her daughter and son-in-law a couple years prior. They were eating a convenient, highly processed diet, and Jeannie found herself simply eating what they did, even though she liked and was used to healthier food. Jeannie relates:

Dr. Nancy gave me a personalized protocol based upon the Ayurveda principles. It included diet, lifestyle changes, when I should eat, and what I should eat, as well as herbal supplements. I had decided after I left her office that I'm going to be absolutely committed to this because I do not want to go down that road that my mother had.

When I came home, I made those changes. I began to follow the diet very closely. I ate a lot of vegetables and grains and also lentils with healthy oils and spices. I also structured my bedtime, which was something that was suggested, and took all the recommended herbal supplements.

Within two weeks' time, I could see a huge difference. I recognized that as I was trying to transpose those numbers in the computer from one place to another, I was remembering them rather than having to write them down. It wasn't difficult to remember words anymore when I was in conversation with family or friends or even in the trainings. I began to see these improvements, and I was going, "This is incredible. This is absolutely incredible." There's been so much change. Even the inflammation in my joints, hip, and knee is way down. It's just remarkable… One other thing is my sleep patterns. Before, I would go to bed 10, 10:30 at night, and I would sleep in the morning as late as anybody, as long as I could. Then I would wake up, and I'd be very groggy, not alert. I used to say, "I might get up at 7, but I'm not awake until about 10," because I just didn't have that alertness.

So I make sure I am always in bed before 10, usually 9 or 9:30. Now I wake up at 5 or 6 without an alarm clock. I'm alert. I'm ready to go for the day, and I'm bright. It's just so different than the patterns that were there before! My mood has changed. I'm much happier, lighter. I laugh more, I'm not as dull, I think. I'm much more lucid all the way across so many parameters in my life. I'm so thrilled!

Needless to say, I was also thrilled to hear Jeannie describe her quick turnaround, especially impressive in just 2 weeks, with diet and sleep habits alone. It confirmed to me once again, the power of the Ayurvedic approach, an entirely unique and complementary dimension to health and healing that I firmly believe everyone can benefit from.

Moreover, Jeannie's bloodwork later revealed a multitude of nutrient and hormone deficiencies that we then set about correcting, but not before her wholesome, home-cooked, anti-inflammatory diet and sleep habits, a la Ayurveda, had already restored health and clarity to her brain and mind.

In summary, the ultimate anti-inflammatory solution is to create *balance*. We need to support robust immunity with healthy diet and lifestyle, while eliminating triggers of excess inflammation. This balance is automatic when we give the body the kind of food, sleep, activity, and pure environment it needs to be healthy and thrive.

Jeannie's recovery demonstrates that we must address inflammation and health throughout the entire body, even when only one organ, like the brain, may be plaguing us. The body, brain, and mind are intimately connected—essentially, they are one. Compartmentalizing is no longer a viable approach to health. For each part to be healthy, the whole must be too.

Common Pathway: Brain and Heart Health

A rapidly growing body of research suggests an intimate link between cardiovascular disease and Alzheimer's. Studies indicate that both conditions co-exist in about 25 to 50 percent of patients, along with common risk factors—including age, hypertension, diabetes, smoking, coronary artery disease, and high cholesterol. The two conditions are so intertwined that their unfavorable effects are more than additive, they're *synergistic*.

One of the key connecting factors in both vascular (blood vessel) disease and Alzheimer's appears to be dysfunction of the blood-brain barrier, which normally keeps the blood and blood-borne factors safely inside the vessels, not seeping into the brain where they can do harm. When this barrier is damaged or "leaky," small proteins and blood cells move out of the blood vessel and into the surrounding brain tissue, stimulating a protective response of amyloid deposition.

This process surrounding leaky blood vessels appears to precede amyloid plaque formation in other parts of the brain and may be one of the antecedent factors that contributes to Alzheimer's disease in the approximately 30 percent of patients with both conditions.

Recent research has found that hypertension, long known as a risk factor for cardiovascular disease, is a risk factor for Alzheimer's disease as well. Even mild elevations in midlife blood pressure matter. An article by Abell et al., published in 2018 in the *European Heart Journal*, reported that mild elevations of systolic blood pressure, as low as 130 at age 50 (but not age 60 or 70), was associated with increased risk of Alzheimer's disease later in life, even in otherwise healthy individuals *without* any cardiovascular disease.

Some *good* news about blood pressure and dementia risk came out recently from the SPRINT Trial, which recruited subjects 50 years old and above, average age 67, with systolic blood pressure of 130 to 180. Subjects were treated "aggressively" with blood pressure medication to achieve a systolic blood pressure below 120. Within 3 years, treated subjects experienced a 19 percent reduced risk of developing MCI (mild cognitive impairment). This reduction was so significant that the trial, planned for 5 years, was stopped after only 3 years to allow this life-saving information to be disseminated and put to use right away.

This good news about treating blood pressure early, and aggressively, squares with the findings of the Harvard Brain Aging Study which reported in *JAMA Neurology* in May 2018 that amyloid and vascular risk are synergistic, in the *bad* way.

Senior author Jasmeer Chhatwal, MD, PhD, put it aptly, with an encouraging slant, "Recent findings suggest elevated brain amyloid is necessary but perhaps not sufficient on its own to predict imminent cognitive decline. … Remarkably, vascular risk appears to be useful in identifying risk of cognitive decline above and beyond a full slate of MRI and PET measures of brain health.

"Perhaps more importantly, we can reduce vascular risk factors through medical treatments and lifestyle interventions and reducing these vascular risk factors might reduce memory loss over time—especially in people with high brain amyloid."

In other words, having vascular risk factors in midlife is a more important predictor of later cognitive decline than burden of amyloid alone, and evidence exists that getting systolic blood pressure below 120 is a very powerful preventive move to get started with.

Now, let's take a quick look at how vascular factors and brain amyloid may be linked in terms of cause via one common pathway—inflammation.

Genetic Predisposition to Inflammation, *and* Late-Onset Alzheimer's

The human immune response is not uniform across individuals, and is strongly influenced by our genetics, which can dramatically affect risk level for Alzheimer's disease. In Chapter One, we mentioned the genetic variant, ApoE4 lipoprotein that tends to promote vigorous inflammation, including in the brain. It also slows down the clearance of amyloid, resulting in excessive loss of neurons and inter-neuronal connections and may accelerate damage to the blood vessels that feed the brain, as well.

On the positive side, the ApoE4 lipoprotein bestows a robust immune response, which may have been an evolutionary advantage when our primate ancestors moved from a clean-living tree habitat to bacteria and parasite-laden life on the ground. Today, however, in our modern, industrialized world, carriers of the gene for ApoE4 can suffer from a wildfire of inflammation as a barrage of modern stress and toxicity constantly challenges the body and overstimulates the immune system.

While the anti-inflammatory, brain-enhancing guidelines in this book are important for all of us, they are especially critical for anyone with one or two copies of the ApoE4 gene. Having 1 copy of the ApoE4 gene can double one's risk of Alzheimer's, and two copies can increase it by as much as twelve-fold.

Keep in mind that these Alzheimer's incidence statistics are based on Americans living the standard, pro-inflammatory American lifestyle and eating the Standard American Diet (SAD). Consequently, they likely grossly overestimate the incidence of Alzheimer's disease among ApoE4 carriers living healthy life-styles. As always, genes are not our destiny, and genes do *not* doom anyone to Alzheimer's.

Rather, adopting an *anti*-inflammatory diet and lifestyle, as outlined in this and subsequent chapters, can dramatically reduce your chances of cognitive decline regardless of your genetics and may very well sharpen your already razor-like mental faculties. The ability to balance our immune systems, and keep our brains healthy, lies in our own hands, now more than ever before.

Inflammation and Your Arteries

Your arteries are responsible for carrying oxygen-rich blood from the heart throughout the body. Their walls are thick and elastic to expand and contract with the blood flow. As we age, cloggy "plaques" can form along the arterial walls, composed of fat, cholesterol, and fibrous tissue that hardens the walls and narrows the arteries. Atherosclerosis, as it's known, leads to strokes, heart attacks, and is an important contributor to Alzheimer's. Inflammation plays a central role in its progression.

Inflammation creates changes in the lining of the arteries, which attract oxidized LDL (the "bad" cholesterol) and immune cells that migrate into the walls of the artery. Once inside the artery wall, these immune cells engulf the LDL, releasing pro-inflammatory molecules called "cytokines," which promote even more inflammation. Essentially, inflammation begets more inflammation. The result is further plaque formation, which is ultimately "capped" by a fibrous coating.

If inflammation continues, tiny inflammatory molecules can weaken the cap designed to hold the plaque in place, making it vulnerable to rupture. Often called the "silent killer," atherosclerosis traditionally shows no symptoms until a plaque ruptures, suddenly clogging the artery and causing a heart attack or stroke. Although atherosclerosis is often considered a heart problem, it can affect arteries anywhere in your body, including the brain.

Women, in particular, are vulnerable to cardiovascular disease in ever-growing numbers. In America alone, one in four women die from heart disease. The most common cause of heart disease in both men and women is narrowing or blockage of the blood vessels that feed the heart itself, causing the chronic chest pain of oxygen deprivation, called "angina," or a sudden, potentially fatal, heart attack.

Disease in the coronary arteries often reflects a bigger problem - widespread arterial disease throughout the body, including the brain. A chronic reduction of blood supply to the brain due to narrowed blood vessels, or an accumulation of small strokes can lead to a type of cognitive decline termed "vascular dementia," which results in direct death of brain cells due to lack of oxygen and blood flow. Early symptoms of vascular type dementia are not usually limited to short-term memory as in typical Alzheimer's but in more widespread deficits in "executive" functions such as judgement, decision-making, organizing, planning and spatial skills.

When atherosclerosis affects the brain, it can result in strokes, along with permanent brain damage as a result from lack of oxygen and interruption or leakage of blood flow to an area of the brain.

Strokes can be small and imperceptible, but accumulate to significant damage over time, contributing to memory loss and further cognitive decline. Strokes can also be sudden and dramatic, leaving a person with a long rehabilitation to regain movement, use of limbs, and sometimes speaking and cognitive ability.

High Blood Pressure

As we've discussed, controlling high blood pressure, or hypertension, in midlife is key to reducing risk of cognitive decline down the line, and control needs to be much tighter than we ever thought before—a systolic blood pressure below 120. With one in three adults in America suffering from high blood pressure, there is a lot of potential for problems, but also now, fortunately, for prevention.

The National Heart, Lung, and Blood Institute classifies blood pressure as follows:

- Normal—below 120/80
- High-normal—120/80 to 139/89
- Stage 1 hypertension—140/90 to 159/99
- Stage 2 hypertension—160/100 or higher

High blood pressure can damage the brain in at least 3 ways.

1. It can promote leakiness of the blood-brain barrier, leading to amyloid deposition in adjacent brain tissue.
2. It can deprive the brain of oxygen and nutrients due to a sudden blockage, a stroke.
3. It can slowly narrow the arteries that supply oxygen-rich blood to the brain, leading eventually to neuronal damage and dementia from chronic lack of nutrients, oxygen and removal of toxins and wastes.

33

While women generally develop high blood pressure 10 years later than men, menopause bestows an increased risk of developing high blood, especially if for those women who are 20 pounds or more overweight or have a family history of the disease. High blood pressure is manageable and preventable by adopting a healthy lifestyle that includes a diet low in salt, sugar, saturated fats, and alcohol.

Physical activity and weight loss are also key factors in lowering your numbers. Research shows that even three short 10-minute walks significantly lowers blood pressure, indicating that even very short intervals of exercise spread through your day can benefit your heart, brain and arteries.

Monitoring Your Blood Pressure

Those at risk, or who already suffer from high blood pressure, should take care to monitor it on an ongoing basis, even once it normalizes, especially if you are relying on diet and exercise alone to keep it under control.

A number of my patients have modified their lifestyles to get their blood pressure down rather than take medication. This can be very successful and ultimately promotes the "whole body health" we are looking for. The caveat is that patients often fall off their exercise and diet programs over time and their blood pressure rises again.

The danger is compounded when blood pressure isn't being monitored and recurrent hypertension goes undetected for months or even years. The bottom line is, you must keep tabs on your blood pressure level, so it doesn't creep up again without your knowing it. If it does, you'll likely incur more damage to your arteries, with higher blood pressure and greater risk of heart attack or stroke as the end result.

If you are unable to lower your blood pressure with diet and exercise, do not discount medication. In my experience, even individuals who are very sensitive to medication can find at least one medication that will lower their blood pressure and not give any noticeable side effects. Find a good internist or cardiologist who will be willing to try you on as many medications as needed until you find the one that will work for you.

I encourage you not to categorically reject medication out of philosophical reasons. I am sharing this from my experience, as most of my patients prefer natural approaches. Unfortunately, my efforts to get reluctant patients to take blood pressure medication when needed have not always been heeded. I have treated all too many patients who made the choice to avoid what they feared would be "unnatural," and ended up with devastating strokes that could have been prevented.

The Two Faces of Cholesterol

Cholesterol is created by the liver and carried in the blood by lipoproteins. We will focus on two main forms; LDL (low-density lipoproteins) and HDL (high-density lipoproteins). Commonly, these cholesterol forms are defined as "bad" and "good," with HDL being the "good" protective cholesterol that absorbs excess cholesterol and carries it back to the liver for processing. Cholesterol is commonly viewed as a "bad guy" to be gotten rid of, since imbalanced levels of it are associated with greater atherosclerosis and heart disease risk.

Yet cholesterol is far from being a villain. Cholesterol is the building block of important hormones such as cortisol, estrogen, and testosterone—and is an essential component of the membrane that surrounds human cells, including brain cells, allowing chemicals to selectively pass in and out of the cell. Balanced cholesterol levels and function are critical to a healthy brain and healthy arteries.

But the "cholesterol equation" is not always as simple as you may have been led to believe. When checking your cholesterol:

35

- Be sure to check your fasting lipid profile, these include the HDL and LDL levels, as well as your total cholesterol level and serum triglycerides.
- Keep your cholesterol in a healthy range—above 150 for brain health, and below 200 to protect your arteries.
- Monitor your LDL particle size and number, as they will indicate how LDL may be affecting your arteries.
- Also, check your blood for lipoprotein(a), often referred to as "lipoprotein little 'a'," a specific inherited protein that can dramatically increase your cardiovascular risk, even in the face of otherwise healthy cholesterol levels.

Also, if your diet falls short of the optimal whole food, anti-inflammatory diet rich in fresh fruits, vegetables and antioxidants, I recommend you check your level of oxidized LDL or "oxyLDL." OxyLDL is a measure of oxidized LDL cholesterol, LDL cholesterol that has been attacked by free radicals and is therefore extra toxic to the body. Notably, LDL does not get laid down in the arterial wall to make plaque unless it is in its oxidized.

Finding out you have elevated levels of oxidized LDL, which puts you at higher risk for heart attack and stroke, just might stimulate you to take action by increasing your intake of antioxidant-rich foods and potentially supplementing your diet with Ayurvedic herbs or other free radical squelching supplements. Although a test not usually covered by insurers, it is an affordable test available through most major laboratories, and also online at self-test sites such as *www.lifeextension.com*.

Stress: The Dark Side of Inflammation

We have clearly seen that inflammation is a two-edged sword. It can save our lives from a life-threatening infection on the one hand or can destroy our health through overactivity on the other hand.

An integral piece of this inflammation dilemma lies in oxidation, the process by which one molecule "steals" an electron from the outer shell of another, making both electrons chemically unstable. More than you wanted to know? The point here is that unstable molecules mix and mingle in a mutually self-destructive way, leading to irreversibly damaged fats, proteins and even DNA—I think you get the picture that this isn't a desirable outcome!

The same process of creating *free radicals* that is destructive to the "bad guy"-- bacteria, viruses, and other invaders—can also be destructive to our own bystander cells when they fall prey to unintended "friendly fire," even as the war on the invader may be being won.

The bottom line is that we need to keep inflammation, *and oxidation,* in check to save our cells, our brains, and our cognition.

No worries, there's some good news in all this. Mother Nature was "on" to it, and in her infinite wisdom, built into our food supply an abundant source of *anti*-oxidants— protective compounds that bind and neutralize excess free radicals— and they're inherent in every fruit, vegetable, herb, spice, coffee bean, tea leaf, legume, nut, and seed. She also gave us abundant enzymes such as SOD, catalase, and *glutathione,* present in every cell, whose primary function is to sop up excess free radicals *before* they attack and damage vital cell components. Oxidation is kept in balance through Mother Nature's antioxidant defense system, both inside and outside of us.

There are many antioxidant supplements on the market today, touted to bestow added protection against free radicals. Vitamins such as C and E, pine bark, and myriad others are all good for you. But there is one virtually undiscovered herbal "supernova" that is important for you to know about. This formula is called Amrit Nectar™.

Amrit Nectar is a traditional Ayurvedic synergistic combo of over three dozen organic herbs, laboriously and meticulously prepared in over 250 steps, in strict accordance with the traditional Ayurvedic texts. This extraordinary care, rare in manufacturing today, is necessary to enliven and protect vital nutrients and ensure maximum potency and effectiveness.

Research indicates this extraordinary diligence in preparing the formula today is fully worth it. Extracts of Amrit Nectar™ tablet ("MAK-4" in studies) have tested out as up to 10,000 times more potent gram per gram than either vitamin C or E, a truly remarkable finding and testament to the intelligence behind its formulation.

The antioxidant ability of Amrit Nectar was demonstrated by its ability to inhibit the oxidation of LDL, the "bad" cholesterol. Blocking LDL oxidation—the necessary first step to arterial plaque formation—is a benefit of great preventive significance. Indeed, in further studies, rabbits who were genetically destined for early heart disease did not get it when liberally fed Amrit Nectar with their standard diet.

Beyond the benefits Amrit Nectar bestows for arterial health, additional research I find particularly exciting involves the impact of Amrit Nectar on the brain, both directly and through its whole-body effects.

Amrit Nectar is rich in some of the most renowned herbs for brain health—including gotu kola and shankapushpi—as well as supportive whole-body herbs for liver, kidney, bowel, immunity, and hormonal balance. So it comes as no surprise that Amrit Nectar has demonstrated a range of beneficial effects in the brain and throughout the body that serve to protect our memory and cognition.

Findings include balancing the immune response, with over-zealous reactions toned down and free radical production likewise tempered. Amrit Nectar directly provides antioxidant protection and also ramps up the brain's *own* antioxidant production, including the key antioxidant enzyme, glutathione, critical to brain health, but often depleted from age, inflammation, and toxin exposure.

Regarding neuronal function, studies indicate that Amrit Nectar enhances acetylcholine production—the neurotransmitter that is the therapeutic target of the major anti-Alzheimer's drugs on the market today. Potentially, taking Amrit Nectar regularly before Alzheimer's sets in may help keep the brain's acetylcholine and antioxidants at optimal levels, another powerful avenue of extra prevention. As with all preventive measures, it's best to start early, *before* serious damage is done.

Even *if* damage is there, one study showed that Amrit Nectar reversed otherwise "irreversible" oxidative damage to brain lipids from free radicals. This remarkable finding was demonstrated in aging guinea pigs, who showed a reduction in the load of "lipofuscin," a pigmented "wear and tear" fat that typically increases as we age. To find that a natural preparation can reverse an otherwise "irreversible" brain aging effect is testament to the healing power that resides within Nature and within ourselves, waiting to be activated.

Keeping our mitochondria strong (the "energy" generators in our cells) is a key factor in anti-aging and maintaining our mental sharpness. In the study above, Amrit Nectar administration also resulted in more youthful levels of oxygen consumption, i.e., *better mitochondrial function*, by brain cells.

A related study showed that 2 months of Amrit actually *reversed* mitochondrial degeneration, as evidenced by repair and restoration of mitochondrial structures, in aging guinea pigs*—a genuine "turning back the clock" finding.

---

* This is not to imply a sanctioning of animal research. In this forum, I seek to share meaningful information I believe may save brains and lives. Harm to life forms of all kinds should be avoided and humane standards for animal participation, according to or exceeding set standards, must be adhered to in all scientific research.

Whereas reduced oxygen consumption due to mitochondria dysfunction shows up as one of the first evidences of impending cognitive decline, (signaling cellular distress, and often followed by amyloid deposition and cognitive decline,) Amrit Nectar notably helps ramp up brain energy production again, reversing the trend of decline.

All in all, studies have demonstrated that Amrti Nectar helps the brain (1) clear out damaged lipids, (2) become more metabolically active, and (3) physically rejuvenate its mitochondria—all exciting and promising findings.

The wide range of effects demonstrated for the brain, nerves, and immune system by the research is quite impressive. Experience of my patients (and my own personal experience) over 30 years is that Amrit Nectar tablet leads to overall greater health, immunity and prevention in a holistic way. If I have to choose one herbal formula only, my "go-to" is Amrit Nectar tablet as it is generally well-tolerated by patients, unlikely to interfere with medications, and supports the overall healing process. Taking a double dose for a time when extra protection is needed often leads to noticeable subjective feelings of greater whole-body strength and integration. From the Ayurvedic point of view, Amrit Nectar tablet is "perfect balance in a jar."

Reversing Heart Disease—Reversing Cognitive Decline

Dr. Dean Ornish established 30 years ago that heart disease can be reversed with diet, lifestyle, meditation, and social support. Just as Dale Bredesen was the first physician to demonstrate that cognitive decline can be reversed without drugs or surgery, Ornish was the first physician to document that heart disease can be halted and even reversed, simply by changing your lifestyle. Based on his landmark, internationally acclaimed study, Ornish's program has helped and inspired countless patients around the world avoid bypass surgery and go on to live healthy, active lives.

In Dr. Ornish's pioneering study, published in 1998, a group of 48 patients with coronary heart disease were randomized to either an intensive lifestyle group, without any lipid-lowering drugs, or a "usual care" group, of moderate lifestyle changes and varying use of lipid-lowering drugs. The intensive lifestyle group followed a very low fat (10 percent) vegetarian diet of whole foods along with aerobic exercise, stress management training, smoking cessation, and group psychosocial support regularly for five years.

The results were stunning. After 5 years, those in the intensive lifestyle group showed a *reversal* of coronary artery narrowing of nearly 8 percent, while the controls had an *increased* narrowing of nearly 30 percent, even though many of them took lipid-lowering medications, while none in the intensive lifestyle group did. Furthermore, the lifestyle group had less than half the number of heart-related events, including heart attacks and hospitalizations compared with the controls.

Over the 5 years of the study, those in the lifestyle group showed cumulative improvement in their lipid levels and atherosclerosis, while the controls—who were given "usual care," and instructed to do moderate exercise—had *progression* of their disease.

This remarkable contrast serves to encourage everyone who aspires to achieve a healthier heart and a better brain, to "take heart." Implement your own lifestyle changes today to protect your blood vessels and your brain and enjoy the rest of your life with full cognitive power and good health.

Calm Your Stress To Squelch Inflammation: Transcendental Meditation

Do you find it hard to get up and get moving? While staying physically active is *necessary and non-negotiable* for heart and brain health, there may be some good news for you about sitting quietly in a chair with your eyes closed. The Transcendental Meditation (TM) technique, which proposes to awaken consciousness and reduce stress, is described as a simple, effortless technique practiced for twenty minutes twice a day while sitting in a comfortable chair. Hundreds of published research studies document its benefits for health, and it just may be one of the most potent heart "medications" you can take.

The TM technique is usually experienced as easy to learn, with results from the start, without requiring many weeks, months or years of practice. During the practice, brain waves shift to a coherent alpha predominance that spreads across the hemispheres, while the mind becomes more settled yet alert, and the body reaches a deep state of rest. Hundreds of peer-reviewed research studies show that TM is effective in reducing stress and anxiety, improving cardiovascular health, and enhancing brain function.

In my clinical practice over several decades, I have noticed that my patients who practice the TM technique regularly in general have a lower incidence of heart disease. Several have remarked that their parents or siblings have been on medication for high blood pressure or had heart attacks, while they themselves remain heart healthy. If they do get high blood pressure, it is usually associated with a strong family history and they develop it years to decades later than others in their family. Indeed, in one sturdy, Orme-Johnson et al. found that practitioners of Transcendental Meditation and Ayurveda together had less than one-tenth the heart disease of age and demographically matched controls.

I have also noticed meditating patients are staying healthy in other ways as they age. Rarely are they on medications, even into their 60s. Findings from a number of research studies sponsored by the NIH and published in journals of the AMA and AHA suggest how the TM technique may support health and longevity by mitigating four key risk factors for inflammation and cognitive decline.

Lower blood pressure. Multiple research studies funded by the NIH and published in American Heart Association journals have shown that regular practice of the TM technique significantly lowers blood pressure, thus preventing damage to the arteries and the brain. In its journal Hypertension, the American Heart Association reported that the Transcendental Meditation technique significantly lowered blood pressure by 10.7 mm Hg and diastolic pressure by 6.4 mm Hg. TM was twice as effective as controls, who practiced muscle relaxation.

Meta-analyses of nearly 30 years of peer-reviewed research supports that TM is at least as effective as exercise and diet for lowering blood pressure—good news for those who prefer to sit and relax over going to the gym! (Although, of course, I say that somewhat in jest, as *everyone* needs to exercise and eat right, no matter what we do to relax.)

Reduced risk of stroke. With reduced blood pressure and thus less stress on the arteries, it makes sense that there would be a reduction in stroke and coronary heart disease, which are both highly correlated with dementia later in life. A 5-year study published in the journal *Circulation* on patients with coronary heart disease, who are at high risk of repeat heart attacks, reported an impressive 48 percent reduction in heart attack, stroke, and death among those practicing the TM technique compared to controls.

TM has also been demonstrated to reduce other risk factors such as atherosclerosis. For instance, a study published in *Stroke* found that people who learned the TM technique showed a reversal of plaque formation as measured by reduced thickness of the carotid artery, after just six months of practice as compared to a health education control group. The control group who received health education on diet and exercise had continued thickening of this artery. This elegant study demonstrates the potential heal-

43

ing power of our minds themselves—a demonstration of "mind-over matter" if there ever was one!

Reduced inflammation. As we have seen, stress is a major contributor to inflammation in the body, and inflammation is one of the key contributors to cognitive decline. In one meta-analysis conducted at Stanford and published in the *Journal of Clinical Psychology*, the Transcendental Meditation technique was found to reduce trait anxiety more effectively than sixteen other self-improvement techniques.

To be more specific, researchers have found that TM reduces stress (sympathetic activity) and increases relaxation (parasympathetic activity). Parasympathetic activity has been shown to have a powerful anti-inflammatory effect. Thus, by reducing stress and promoting parasympathetic activity, TM practice promotes an anti-inflammatory effect throughout the body.

Another study that points to the anti-inflammatory benefits of TM found reduced periodontal inflammation in TM practitioners. It is now known that there is a strong connection between gum disease and heart disease. In other words, reduced inflammation in the gums is an indication of reduced inflammation in the cardiovascular system and the rest of the body.

Balanced blood sugar levels. Due to our nation's high-carbohydrate diet and lack of exercise, there has been an upsurge in glycotoxicity (blood sugar regulation problems) in American women, especially as they age. The toxic, pro-inflammatory effect of excess glucose on the brain results in a chronic reduction in the brain's insulin response a condition known as insulin resistance. When the brain stops responding, insulin levels drop, causing impaired brain functioning. Insulin has a beneficial, trophic effect, causing brain cells to grow. Without it, brain cells atrophy and die at a faster rate.

In a 2006 study published in *JAMA,* the Transcendental Meditation™ technique has been shown to decrease metabolic syndrome and improve insulin sensitivity and blood sugar control, as compared to controls, thus preventing damage to the brain.

How To Listen To Your Body

The body has its own infinite intelligence. If you listen to your body, you are listening to a bigger and more comprehensive intelligence that can guide you to do what is best for you. For this, you need to become more self-aware. Just putting a little attention on yourself can go a long way. For example, you can ask yourself: "Does this make me feel good?" If I sleep for 8 hours, I feel great. If I sleep for 4 hours, I feel terrible. If I eat that food, I feel fantastic, but if I overeat some midnight snacks, I'm going to have congestion and aches the next day. This is how you start to learn what is best for you, from yourself, because everything is right here within you. You just need to pay attention.

Align your routine with nature's rhythms and cycles (see Chapter Five for more details) and you can transform your body to feel more energized, be more productive, and ultimately feel like the best possible version of yourself. Keep a journal, which can help you note changes in your body on a daily, weekly, and monthly basis. Track your energy levels, moods, and sleep quality—as well as blood pressure, blood sugar, or any other parameter of interest—in relation to certain foods, bedtime, exercise, and mealtimes to identify and master the ideal diet, routine, and lifestyle that is right for you.

Conventional Therapies

Aspirin Therapy

Before menopause, women have a lower risk of heart attack than men of the same age. This benefit disappears after about 10 years post-menopause. Eventually, women have a higher risk of hypertension and stroke than men. For women who are identi-

45

fied as being at increased risk of stroke, a baby aspirin has been shown to provide some protection. It is important to note that aspirin can damage the stomach lining, promote GI bleeding, increase hemorrhagic stroke or lead to leaky gut syndrome. Take aspirin only if your doctor recommends it.

Statin Therapy

Statins are a popular class of drugs for lowering cholesterol levels in the blood, as well as reducing inflammation, which may be how it exerts its primary anti-heart attack effects. However, statins can be a double-edged sword. For optimal brain health, you have to make sure that your cholesterol does not get too low. A cholesterol level below 150 may adversely affect cognition. The brain needs cholesterol to make many protective components of the nervous system. Patients have presented to me with symptoms of depression, memory loss, and insomnia that cleared gradually after restoring their cholesterol to a more optimal level—not too high and not too low.

Doctors can recommend statin therapy too readily, in my opinion, often beyond the official guidelines for prescribing. Three of the main appropriate indications for statin therapy include:

- You have had a heart attack, stroke, or peripheral vascular disease.
- You have diabetes.
- You have a 7.5 percent chance of having a heart attack or stroke within the next 10 years.

To assess your risk, I recommend you calculate it using the MESA calculator at *www.mesa-nhlbi.org/MESACHDRisk/ MesaRiskScore/RiskScore.aspx*. If your risk is less than 7.5 percent, you do not have any of the other risk factor above, and your doctor is still recommending a statin, bring it up as a discussion.

Statins are a potent medication and should only be used if really necessary.

Some of my patients who refuse statins have been willing to take Red Yeast Rice, which contains a naturally occurring statin called "lovastatin." This is the most effective supplement I have found that predictably lowers cholesterol, and patients rarely report side effects. Do check with your doctor before starting it to be sure there is no contraindication and stop taking it immediately and alert her if you experience any side effects. Also, make sure you take a brand that is tested for authenticity, purity, and has standardized active ingredients. The website *www.consumerlab.com* is a reliable resource for quality control information on most supplements on the market and provides good value for its nominal membership fee.

How To Keep Inflammation In Check, *Naturally*

The vigor and balance of our immune system depends on our overall level of health. The ultimate inflammatory challenge is to create *balance*—maintaining robust immune protection, while eliminating triggers of excess inflammation. This balance is automatic when we give our bodies the kind of food, sleep, activity, and pure environment they need to be healthy and thrive. Let's look at some of the actions you can take to keep your immunity strong and your inflammation in line.

Tomassina's Story: Proof of Purity

Tomassina is a 57-year-old, newly retired law enforcement officer from New York City, whose internist had been advising for years to take a statin for her mildly elevated cholesterol. She had resisted, out of concern for side effects, and the fact that she was overall in excellent health without any other risk factors for heart attack or stroke. Yet, on her own, she hadn't been able to get it down, even with changes in diet and a long habit of walking several miles a day.

Tomassina came to see me when she visited The Raj Ayurveda Health Spa to gently de-stress and detox her body from years of an intense career and thousands of miles walking her beat and breathing exhaust-filled city air. She told me about her desire to lower her cholesterol without statins and was willing to change her diet, eat mainly home-cooked meals, and take herbs after returning home. I designed an individualized program for her based on her unique Ayurvedic constitution and imbalances.

Two months after her treatment at The Raj, Tomassina wrote to me, ecstatic. Her cholesterol had dropped dramatically, to an absolutely ideal number, which she attributed to the "Ayurvedic herbal detox diet" and her detox treatment at The Raj. Her total cholesterol went from 237 in May of that year to 165 now, six months later. Her LDL (the "bad cholesterol") went from 157 to 96. Her doctor was impressed and, given her perfect readings, rightfully agreed that she no longer needed a statin. Tomassina continues to enjoy her Ayurvedic lifestyle, feels very satisfied from her Ayurvedic anti-inflammatory diet rich in organic, whole foods, herbs and spices and is committed to keeping her cholesterol in the healthy range, without a statin.

Spice It Up for a Healthy Heart

Spices are beginning to assume their rightful medicinal role as a concentrated source of antioxidants, immune-boosters, and anti-inflammatories. Herbs and spices, the penultimate "food as medicine," are no longer destined to get old, stale, and collect dust in our kitchen cabinets. (How many of us have years-old spice bottles in our cupboards? Throw them out and get fresh ones—they lose their potency within a few months of opening.)

Thousands of recent research studies are proving beyond a doubt that spices have potent medicinal effects and point to the value of including them every day in our meals and cooking. Spices are rich in a variety of phytochemicals that can help prevent illness and disease. The following spices have been shown to be beneficial to heart and brain health.

Turmeric	Turmeric is a strong antioxidant that reduces inflammation, prevents amyloid and atherosclerotic plaque buildup, and lowers the chances of a heart attack.
Cardamom	Cardamom is high in magnesium and zinc and helps to lower blood pressure and inflammation.
Garlic	Garlic has a powerful compound called allicin that may lower your chance of heart disease, helps moderate blood pressure, and can lower cholesterol.
Ginger	Ginger supports beneficial intestinal bacteria, promotes good digestion, and has strong antioxidant and anti-inflammatory elements that may help prevent heart disease.
Cinnamon	Cinnamon has documented abilities to lower blood sugar, reduce inflammation, and fend off cell-damaging free radicals. Helps the body metabolize carbohydrates.

Diet

Research has found that consumption of a wholesome Mediterranean-like diet high in plant-based foods, healthy fats, and spices led to a significant positive change in immune function and is anti-inflammatory. Here are some benefits and guidelines to help you begin to eat the healthy, delicious Mediterranean way.

Mediterranean Diet Benefits

Research has shown that the traditional Mediterranean diet reduces the risk of heart disease. The Mediterranean diet caused reductions in oxidized LDL cholesterol, the "bad" cholesterol, along with improvements in several other heart disease risk factors. In fact, a meta-analysis of more than 1.5 million healthy adults demonstrated that following a Mediterranean diet was associated with a reduced risk of cardiovascular mortality as well as overall mortality.

The Mediterranean diet is also associated with a reduced incidence of cancer, Parkinson's and Alzheimer's diseases. Researchers found that eating a Mediterranean diet slows some changes in the brain that may indicate early Alzheimer's disease. Women who eat a Mediterranean diet supplemented with extra-virgin olive oil and mixed nuts may have a reduced risk of breast cancer. For these reasons, it is highly recommended for healthy adults to adapt a style of eating like that of the Mediterranean diet for prevention of major inflammatory, chronic diseases.

When I create a dietary plan for patients, I see one-on-one, I may also incorporate or even build their dietary plan around Ayurvedic principles. As with Jeannie, who healed her brain in two weeks with an anti-inflammatory, "Ayurvedic" vegetarian diet personalized for her, you may also benefit from adopting Ayurvedic diet and eating principles. Check out the "digestive type" quiz at *www.drnancyhealth.com* and get weekly tips for your type that will help you incorporate those Ayurvedic practices most likely to benefit you.

Mediterranean Diet Principles

What we call the Mediterranean diet is derived from the traditional eating and social patterns of the regions around the Mediterranean such as southern Italy, Greece, Turkey, and Spain. The Mediterranean diet is not a diet, as in "go on a diet," even though it can be a great way to lose weight or improve your health. Rather, it is a lifestyle—including foods, activities, and meals with friends and family. Generally, people in these regions spend a lot of time outdoors in nature; eat together with family and friends (rather than alone or on-the-go); and put aside time to laugh, dance, garden, and practice hobbies.

The Mediterranean diet emphasizes eating primarily organic, non-GMO, unprocessed plant-based foods such as fruits and vegetables, whole grains, legumes, and nuts. This diet replaces butter with healthy fats such as olive oil and uses herbs and spices instead of salt to flavor foods.

Eating *fresh, organic, non-GMO* foods is a sure way to keep you healthier as you avoid accumulating damaging toxins, herbicides and pesticides, all of which can directly harm the brain and other systems in your body.

In the table below, you'll find suggested foods to include as you eat "the Mediterranean way."

You should also avoid sugar, refined grains such as white bread, pasta made with refined wheat, trans fats found in margarine and various processed foods, refined oils such as soybean oil, canola oil, cottonseed oil, processed meat, and any highly processed foods.

Fruits (preferably in season)	Apples, bananas, berries, cherries, cantaloupe, plums, pears, peaches, oranges, etc.
Vegetables (non-starchy)	Leafy greens like spinach and kale, asparagus, zucchini, broccoli, eggplant, cauliflower, artichokes, tomatoes, carrots, green beans, fennel. (Note: The USDA and other health-focused organizations recommend adult women eat 2½ cups of vegetables per day and 3 cups for men; and dark leafy veggies several times a week. The Duke Diet and Exercise Center in North Carolina ranked dark leafy greens as the most nutrient dense food.)
Vegetables (starchy)	In small quantity: sweet potatoes, winter squash.
Whole grains	Rice, whole wheat. (Note: Since gluten sensitivity and high glycemic rice can be an issue, I usually recommend small amounts of quinoa, amaranth, and possibly occasional brown basmati or organic wild rice instead. See Chapter Four for further help in assessing and optimizing your carb intake and blood sugar.)

Legumes	Lentils of all kinds, chickpeas. (Note: I would also add mung bean dahl, whole or split, which is a good source of protein with one of the lowest contents of anti-nutrients. Be sure to soak all lentils and other legumes in water overnight. Ayurveda also recommends dry roasting them in a pan before cooking and adding lemon during cooking to further enhance digestibility.)
Nuts and seeds	Almonds (blanched is best), sesame seeds, cashews, pistachios, walnuts. (Note: Ayurveda recommends soaking nuts to make them lighter and easier to digest. The firm texture of raw almonds makes them hard to digest, as per study published in *Food Biophysics* in 2009. Also, soaking removes the tannins and phytates which humans cannot digest. For more information see *https://lilynicholsrdn.com/why-eating-nuts-upsets-yourstomach/*.)
Oils	"Extra-virgin" and "virgin" olive oils.
Spice and fresh herbs	Basil, oregano, fresh mint, pepper, garlic.
Drink	Plenty of fresh water, herbal teas. (Alcohol is not recommended for optimizing brain health.)
Fish	Fatty, cold water fish, including wild caught mackerel (not king mackerel), lake trout, herring, sardines, anchovies, and salmon (the "SMASH" fish, plus lake trout) are rich sources of omega-3 fatty acids.

Anti-inflammatory, Omega-3 Fatty Acid Supplements for Your Brain

From an anatomical point of view, we are all "fat-heads." Curiously, our brains are composed of fully 60 percent fat! Fat is a major component of every cell membrane in the brain, and particularly important to the long axons that conduct signals across brain regions and to our *protective* neurons, our glial cells. Needless to say, a diet lacking in fat is not good for our brains, and, according to Ayurveda, leads to excess "dryness," a risk factor for atrophy and degeneration.

Within the family of healthy fats for our brains and health as a whole, the omega-3 essential fatty acids, named for their particular molecular structure, play a key role. They build all cell membranes, reduce inflammation, balance blood sugar, and increase the activity of BDNF, a key brain molecule, which stimulates new cell growth. In doing so, they are critical to normal, balanced mood, memory, and overall brain functioning. Low levels of omega-3 fats have been linked to dementia as well as depression, anxiety, ADHD, mood swings, and bipolar disorder.

While both types of the essential fatty acids—omega-6 and omega-3—are important for health, omega-6s, which are pro-inflammatory, are the most abundant in our modern diets, while the anti-inflammatory omega-3s, which come in two major forms, DHA and EPA, are consumed in less quantity. This sets up an imbalance favoring inflammation that we must take measures to correct.

I would estimate that four out of every five patients I test are on the wrong side of the omega-6:omega-3 balance. As a result, I end up recommending omega-3 supplementation to almost every brain patient I see—whether for treatment or prevention. (Exceptions include patients on blood thinners, with a bleeding tendency, or with a type of amyloidosis of cerebral blood vessels, as omega-3s can "thin" the blood at higher doses.)

The omega-3 fatty acid most plentiful in the brain is DHA, which is a critical component of synapses, the membranous ends of neurons where communication between neurons takes place. Numerous studies have shown that DHA supports synaptic health, a key factor in memory and cognition. At least one clinical trial has found that supplementing with DHA resulted in significant improvement in cognitive function in older subjects with mild cognitive impairment. In this study, research subjects were given 900 mg of DHA daily, and showed measurable improvements in learning and memory at the end of 6 months. The authors suggest that longer-term studies may reveal an even greater cognitive improvement over time in those with memory impairment, as well as a potential *preventive* effect that has yet to be documented in cognitively healthy seniors.

Most omega-3 fats come from *wild* plants, animals, and fish. Not so easy to find these days. Most people being deficient in omega-3s, it is important to support your omega-3 fat intake with targeted foods and supplements. Fish oil is a good source of omega-3's but be sure you choose a brand that vouches for its purity through laboratory testing for PCBs and heavy metals. Also, store in a cool, dark place such as your refrigerator since fish oil can go rancid very easily, taking on toxic, rather than beneficial, effects.

Other sources of omega-3s:

- Wild-caught, cold-water fish such as wild salmon and sardines are best. (Small fish and small quantities are safest, to minimize mercury contamination. Avoid farm-raised fish, where small, purer fish are often fed bigger, toxic fish in a reversal of the normal food chain, making small fish toxic too!)
- DHA for ApoE4: Emerging research indicates for ApoE4 positive individuals absorb essential fatty acids (especially DHA) best from krill oil (a small crustacean), fish eggs or whole fish. DHA in these products is present in a phospholipid form which enters the brain more readily in ApoE4 conditions. Regular, non-phospholipid DHA/fish oil doesn't get into the brain well in older individuals with ApoE4, likely due to damage to the blood-brain barrier.
- Organic, omega-3 eggs, also a good source of choline, needed for our brain to make acetylcholine, a major memory neurotransmitter.

- Flax, hemp, and soaked nuts such as walnuts, almonds, and pecans. (These foods contain a form of omega-3 that must undergo transformation in the body before it becomes usable. As we get older, our ability to do this drops. My recommendation is to, of course, eat a diet rich in nuts and seeds, but also consider taking a pure, safety-tested omega-3 supplement, especially DHA, on a regular basis.)

The Importance of the Omega-6:Omega-3 Ratio

While our ancestors enjoyed a diet with a balanced 1:1 ratio of omega-6 to omega-3 essential fatty acids, the average American today consumes a diet of as much as 12:1 to 25:1. This means we are taking in 12 to 14 times the amount of omega-6s as we evolved to handle. An excess of omega-6 in the diet, without enough anti-inflammatory omega-3 to balance it out, can lead to excess inflammation in the body, and brain, which of course is to be avoided. To feed your brain, try to maintain a 1:1 ratio or higher in favor of omega-3s.

Testing the omega-6:omega-3 ratio in your blood is the best way to know where you stand in the omega fatty acid arena. Your ratio should be less than 3. However, it should not fall below 0.5 to avoid increasing the risk of hemorrhage.

Exercise

Sitting for long periods of time is associated with increased deposition of fat around the heart and clogging of the arteries, even in those who exercise regularly outside of their time at work. It is also linked to atrophy of brain regions having to do with memory. One strategy to counter hours being glued to your desk chair is to get up every 25 minutes or so and walk around for a few minutes. Apps like Pomodoro can help you keep track of time. I'm a great believer in standing desks, which I use myself every day, and can reduce your total sitting time while promoting greater alertness and productivity.

In addition, regular exercise and staying fit is essential to both heart health and cognition. The generally recommended amount is 30 to 60 minutes most days of the week. The Harvard Men's Health Watch, 2015, recommends interval exercise, which confers added benefits for weight loss and fitness level and consists of short bursts of faster exercise alternating with slower paced intervals of recovery. For example, walking as fast as you can for 1 to 2 minutes is followed by a leisurely pace for the same amount of time, then fast walking is repeated. In general, exercise promotes growth hormones, helps with weight loss, burns calories, improves mood, increases blood flow, and keeps your channels clear. We'll explore exercise further in Chapter Six.

Sleep

Getting optimal sleep is also key to keeping inflammation in check, our minds and memory sharp, and heart disease at bay. The ideal is to sleep at least 6 and up to 8 hours every night. Less than 6 hours of sleep doubles the risk of heart attack and stroke, while more than 8 hours increases angina and coronary artery disease. After age 60, the risks associated with sleep deprivation become even greater. The timing of sleep is also a factor, with night owls at higher risk. We'll dive into additional fascinating details about optimal sleep habits in Chapter Six.

Five "Do's" for Your Heart

1. Create balance in your life through wholesome, whole foods-based diet, and adjust your diet and routine according to your body's cues and feedback.
2. Eat the Mediterranean way, and avoid sugar, refined carbs, processed foods, cigarettes, and excess alcohol.

3. Learn and practice Transcendental Meditation or a stress-relieving technique of your choice on a daily basis.
4. Get 6 to 8 hours of sleep per night.
5. Stay physically active.

What Tests To Do

The Next Step: Now it's ideal to find out your own level of inflammation, and if elevated, what may be making your body react. Beyond protecting your brain, greater longevity and improved overall health are expected side-benefits.

Testing gives an objective measure of how your immune system is working, and if excess inflammation is an issue. I firmly believe that knowing your level of inflammation, by a variety of markers, is an important step in evaluating your risk for cognitive decline, and an important motivator if you discover your inflammatory response is dangerously out of line. Remember, you *can* correct this, and, barring specific medical conditions, usually without drugs and their side-effects. When testing for inflammation, be sure to check the following markers. While not an exhaustive list, it is a reasonable, affordable place to start:

hs-CRP (high-sensitivity C-reactive protein): This is a protein that the liver makes when there is inflammation in the body. It is a strong marker of inflammation in the blood that predicts arterial inflammation, cancer, infection, and heart disease. It can be temporarily elevated due to an acute infection or injury, so be sure to repeat the test a few months later if you think that may apply to you. A high level of hs-CRP, if caused by an immune reaction to environmental factors, can usually be reduced through a healthy diet and exercise regime.

TGF-beta1 (transforming growth factor-beta 1): A measure of chronic activation of the immune response and a surrogate marker for exposure to biotoxins.

Homocysteine: This is a metabolic byproduct that builds up when B vitamins (folate, B12, B6) or methylation sources are inadequate. Homocysteine is pro-inflammatory and associated with increased risk of heart disease, stroke, osteoporosis, and dementia. Usually correctable with B vitamins in their "methyl-" form. Those with poor methylation ability caused by genetics may need to supplement their diets with betaine, TMG, or other methyl sources as well. (Check your methylation ability with a "MTHFR" test through LabCorp or other standard laboratories. If you have genetic results from *www.23andme.com*, you may upload them to *www.geneticgenie.com* for a report of your gene type for MTHFR as well as many more detoxification enzymes.)

Omega-6:Omega-3 ratio: An optimal level ensures your essential fatty acid balance is helping to keep inflammation in check, not promoting it. Available at standard labs and online for self-testing.

How to Assess Your Artery Health (Additional Optional Tests)

To accurately understand the health of your arteries, consider taking the following evaluations:

MESA (The Multi-Ethnic Study of Atherosclerosis) offers an online risk calculator that can calculate your 10-year risk of coronary heart disease. You will need to know your total cholesterol, HDL cholesterol, and your systolic blood pressure.

The MESA calculator is most accurate if you also include your "coronary artery calcium score" when you enter your data. If you have a family history of heart disease, or have high blood pressure, diabetes, or other risk factors for heart disease, ask your doctor to order a "coronary artery calcium score" test for you.

This test involves a specialized, "ultrafast," low-dose computerized tomography (CT) scan of the heart that measures the amount of calcium in the walls of the arteries, a surrogate measure of atherosclerotic plaque. The test is relatively inexpensive, as low as $100 when self-pay, and gives objective data to calculate your future risk of developing coronary artery disease.

Carotid ultrasound: This non-invasive measure will reveal any significant buildup of plaque in the main arteries in the neck that carry oxygen-rich blood to your brain. While your doctor can order it for you, insurance does not always cover it for screening purposes. It is available inexpensively through mobile, direct-to-consumer testing programs such as *www.lifelinescreening.com*. Check online for scheduled visits to your area.

Take This Simple Action #2 Now!

Go to *www.thehealthybrainsolution.com/lifestyle* and take the short lifestyle quiz to see how well your diet and lifestyle are preventing, or promoting, optimal brain health. You'll get highly doable, personalized tips based on your answers.

www.thehealthybrainsolution.com/lifestyle

3

Heal Your Gut to Heal Your Brain

All disease begins in the gut.

—Hippocrates

Key #3: Heal Your Gut and Better Your Brain

Most of us give nary a thought to our digestive process, unless of course it calls out to us with stomach pains, gas, bloating, heartburn, constipation, or other uncomfortable symptoms. On the medical side, I've observed that digestion is the "furthest thing" from my physician colleagues' minds when addressing any number of "non-gut" issues, such as arthritis, autoimmune disorders, chronic fatigue, anxiety, depression and even, ironically, gastrointestinal diseases including ulcerative colitis and Crohn's disease. "Diet has nothing to do with your condition," patients report their specialists saying, and the digestive process is never even considered, presumed to be "normal."

Fortunately, this blind eye to gut health is changing rapidly. Conventional medicine is beginning to realize that the health of our digestive system is key to our whole-body health. As Hippocrates, the father of western medicine, once said, "all disease begins in the gut." Ayurveda, as well, has long held that food is our best medicine and real healing starts with establishing good digestion.

Current scientific research is revealing the pivotal role our GI tract plays in nearly every aspect of our health. The gut's seminal role is mediated via two vast, interacting networks that until recently have been wholly unappreciated: first, our gut's nervous system of over 500 million neurons and second, its sophisticated population of over 39 trillion hard-working bacteria, more than the total number of cells in our bodies (estimated at 37.2 trillion human cells).

Research has begun to uncover a tremendous amount of "cross-talk" going on between our brains and our guts at every moment. Indeed, our gut and perhaps most significantly, our gut *bacteria*, are conversing with our brains, influencing hormone production, metabolic function, neurotransmitter balance, and perhaps most importantly, immunity and levels of inflammation in both gut and brain. Much of this conversation is occurring through tiny molecules called "metabolites," carried in the blood, mainly from gut to brain. These same metabolites can promote inflammation in the brain, a key process in Alzheimer's disease, and therefore of much interest to researchers today.

Much Ado About BBB: The Blood-Brain Barrier

Our brains rely on a tight barrier between the blood and its own tissue. Progressively smaller and smaller blood vessels carry oxygen and nutrient-rich blood to the brain, ending in our tiniest vessel, the capillary. Capillary walls are composed of a single layer of cells tightly woven together, precisely to keep blood cells and large molecules in, while letting only the smallest nutrients and oxygen out. An "intact," healthy blood-brain barrier is instrumental in maintaining a healthy brain. As we saw in Chapter Two, an inflamed blood-brain barrier can "leak" unwanted molecules into the brain tissue, inciting an inflammatory reaction in and around the vessel, resulting in the deposition of decidedly unwelcome amyloid plaque.

It turns out that our gut and gut bacteria play a huge role in the health of our blood-brain barrier. We'll take a closer look at that, and the fascinating knowledge of how to heal our gut and seal our blood-brain barrier, later in this chapter.

Now, let's consider our very intelligent gut's own "brain" and how it connects to the brain in our heads.

Gut Smart

Dubbed our "second brain" by Justin and Erica Sonnenburg, PhDs, in their acclaimed book *The Good Gut*, the GI tract houses some 500 million neurons, five times more than the number of neurons in the human spinal cord. These neurons, our "enteric nervous system," span the distance from mouth to anus, and profoundly influence our bodies and our brains. The enteric nervous system communicates with the brain via more than thirty different neurotransmitters that pass along nerves or enter the circulation that feeds the brain.

Our digestive system even plays an intimate role in our moods, memory, and thought processes. Currently, more than 90 percent of our serotonin (a neurotransmitter responsible for feelings of well-being and happiness, that most antidepressants today act to increase) and 50 percent of our body's dopamine (another neurotransmitter that sparks motivation, addiction, and reward-driven behavior as well as positive mood) is manufactured in our guts.

The digestive system sports a direct connection to the brain via the vagus nerve, a bi-directional highway that helps control the automatic functioning of the heart, lungs, and digestive tract, commanding unconscious body processes such as heart rate, breathing, and digestion. The vagus nerve is the longest autonomic nerve in the entire body. Interestingly, a full 90 percent of its nerve fibers are dedicated to sending messages regarding your internal organs *from* the gut *to* the brain, with over 400 times the number of messages going up to the brain than the brain sends back to the body. This highlights the tremendous importance our brain and overall body intelligence puts on what is going on in the gut. Gut health is key to brain health. For a healthy brain, we have to make and keep our guts healthy. In today's world, that is a lifelong endeavor, with no better time to start than now.

Gut Bacteria and Our Immunity

While the nervous system of the gut is intimate to our moods, emotions, hormones, and brain function, it is also critical to factor in the central role that our gut bacteria, our "microbiome," play in gut health and gut-brain interaction. The microbiome is getting tremendous attention today, and for good reason.

Our microbiome consists of trillions of beneficial bacteria, commensal (neutral), and pathogenic (detrimental) bacteria—along with incidental fungi, and viruses—that participate in nearly every function of the human body. The microbiome works to produce nutrients, modulates immunity, signals the body to begin detoxifying functions, and influences neurotransmitters as well as hormones.

Perhaps most importantly, the gut's estimated 39 to 100 trillion bacteria interact intimately with the immune system, a full 70 percent of which is housed in the gut. This intimate microbiome-immune connection modulates whether a disease is kept at bay or is facilitated, as in autoimmune conditions.

When healthy, our gut bacteria support proper nutrient digestion and absorption, mood, hormonal balance, and detoxification, essentially communicating "health" to the immune system and brain. However, our gut microbes are in a precarious balance that can be easily upset by improper diet, stress, and antibiotics, all of which most of us get too much of. When our digestive system falls under duress, we are vulnerable to a myriad of symptoms, including fatigue, gas and bloating, hair, skin, nail issues, weight gain, and brain fog, to name a few. If imbalance continues, frank illnesses may result, including allergies, asthma, arthritis, autoimmune conditions, and even potentially cancer, heart disease, and Alzheimer's.

When Things Go Wrong

The Microbiome and Your Brain

In the *Journal of Medicinal Food*, researcher Leo Galland explains that gut microbes shape the architecture of sleep, hormones, and stress reactivity of the hypothalamic-pituitary-adrenal axis—how we react to stress. They influence memory, mood, and cognition and are clinically relevant to a range of disorders, including alcoholism, chronic fatigue syndrome, fibromyalgia, and restless legs syndrome. As the bacteria in our gut synthesize and help balance our hormones and neurotransmitters, changes in our microbiome from poor diet or the introduction of antibiotics, can directly affect how we feel and behave emotionally and physically.

In a study done on mice, it was discovered that when the microbiome is compromised by a course of antibiotics, the mice had substantially higher concentrations of their major stress hormone corticosterone (the human equivalent is cortisol), which negatively impacts memory and reduces BDNF, a protein that stimulates neurogenesis and synaptic growth—both necessary for healthy learning and memory.

The take-home here is that a seemingly innocuous course of antibiotics, for a urinary tract infection (UTI) for example, may leave us forgetful and even depressed.

For example, after a series of UTIs over the course of a year and two rounds of antibiotics, my patient Elouise, at 72 years old, wondered why she felt seriously depressed for the first time in her adult life. After a concerted effort to rebuild her gut microbiome and preventive measures to avert further UTIs (including the nutritional supplements cranactin and D-mannose, and vaginal hormones), Elouise returned to her usual cheerful self, and has continued to feel well, and is UTI-free, 3 years later.

As an aside, recurrent UTIs are frequent in post-menopausal women, as the vaginal tissue thins, protective flora may dwindle, and bacteria more easily ascend to the bladder via the urethra. UTIs can have a major impact on our brains (even before antibiotic treatment) and are a common cause of acute memory loss and confusion (usually reversible) in elderly women. By way of prevention, vaginal hormones can help "plump" the tissues again, and imbalanced flora can be tested for and corrected for additional protection.

To summarize, an unhealthy gut, including compromised flora (imbalanced bacteria), can lead to too many or too few hormones being produced in the body. When the body makes too little serotonin, we begin to feel depressed; too much estrogen and we have difficulty regulating our glucose levels; not enough dopamine and we may feel bored yet low in motivation.

Our neuroendocrine systems secrete hormones according to complex interactions between gut and brain, modulating our emotions, our hormones, and our brain function moment-to-moment. Attending to our gut health turns out to be one of the best ways we can feel better, think sharper, and protect our brain health for the long run.

Inflammation and Alzheimer's

Currently, it is believed that chronic inflammation of the brain plays an essential role in neurodegeneration. While it is unclear whether this inflammation is confined to isolated brain regions or occurs throughout the brain, inflammation in general is seen in patients with Alzheimer's disease, particularly affecting the white matter of the brain (the connecting tracts) and the blood-brain barrier.

Like the gut, the brain is protected by a barrier that controls what enters it from the blood. This blood-brain barrier relies on the integrity of a single layer of cells that lets in oxygen, nutrients, and hormones while it blocks out anything that may cause harm. When this protective layer of endothelial cells is compromised, as happens with inflammation, the brain becomes vulnerable to damage.

The disruption of the blood-brain barrier due to inflammation, postulated in Alzheimer's disease, can allow autoantibodies to cross the blood-brain barrier and attack neurons, resulting in further inflammation, cell death, and the formation of amyloid plaques, all further promoting the neuro-degenerative changes of Alzheimer's disease.

In one groundbreaking study done on mice in the early stages of Alzheimer's disease, researchers focused on gut bacteria rather than directly on brain matter, in an attempt to reduce inflammatory factors, metabolites, and hormones that adversely affect the blood-brain barrier.

The researchers were able to show that modulating gut microbes positively affected communication from gut to brain via the vagus nerve and resulted in a slowing of Alzheimer's disease progression. Their work suggests that changing the composition of the gut microbiome can reduce inflammation and result in improved cognitive function—opening up a whole new avenue for the prevention and treatment of cognitive decline.

Leaky Gut Syndrome

Increased intestinal permeability, commonly termed "leaky gut," is a condition where the lining of the small intestine becomes damaged, loosening the spaces between cells and causing undigested food particles, toxic waste products, and bacteria to enter the blood stream. The gut barrier is comprised of a single layer of epithelial cells and is the most extensive mucosal surface of the body. The cells that make up the barrier are linked together with tight junctions that protect your intestinal walls from allowing unintended molecules from entering the blood.

Tight junctions between your gut cells maintain the delicate balance between allowing vital nutrients to enter your blood-stream, while remaining small enough to prevent undigested particles from passing from your digestive system into the rest of your body.

Therefore, leaky gut, and all its potential health conse-quences, results from malfunction of the intestinal tight-junction proteins. When the tight junctions get "loose," undigested food particles, microorganisms, and toxins can enter the blood stream. What ensues are unhealthy inflammatory, immunological, auto-immune, and neoplastic (cancer-causing) reactions, which, over time, can lead to a wide range of health concerns. Increased intes-tinal permeability has been demonstrated to be a factor in several diseases, such as Crohn's disease, celiac, diabetes, arthritis, cer-tain types of cancer, and others.

Leaky gut is often caused by diet, especially allergies to com-monly consumed foods such as gluten, soy, or dairy, as well as alcohol consumption. Notably, even one episode of binge drink-ing can render an otherwise healthy gut "leaky" for days.

It is now understood that the extensive damage to liver, gut, and brain from chronic alcohol use ensues, at least in part, from inflammation and leakiness of the gut lining. Other proven triggers of leaky gut include medications such as antibiotics, steroids, aspirin, NSAIDs and acetaminophen. These drugs can irritate and inflame the intestinal lining, damage the protective layers and lead to increased intestinal permeability.

Studies have found that in those who suffer from celiac dis-ease (a genetically determined gluten allergy), gluten consump-tion sets off an immune reaction that weakens the intercellular

68

tight junctions and often manifests in symptoms such as diarrhea, headaches, fatigue, and joint pain.

However, gluten consumption can trigger leaky gut in many more people than those genetically susceptible to gluten. Non-celiac gluten intolerance may lead to similar symptoms, or none, as I've found in some patients. In these cases, gluten is a "silent disruptor," resulting in antibody formation by the gut lining cells (as evidenced by gluten antibodies in saliva samples, for example,) even without the celiac gene or antibodies in the blood, a more advanced stage of immune reaction.

I highly recommend you test yourself for gluten allergy, including a saliva antibody sample along with more conventional blood and genetic testing. Avoiding gluten is important with any positive result, as immune reaction against gluten is associated with increased risk of dementia if one continues to consume it. Antibodies mean inflammation, and we know we have to keep that in check, especially in the gut and the brain, to stay sharp and brain-healthy.

Unfortunately, as many as one-third of individuals living in Western society have leaky gut, as defined by increased blood levels of bacterial endotoxin (highly inflammatory cell wall fragments) following intake of a high-fat, high-calorie meal "trigger."

Indeed, in a landmark study from the University of North Texas, McFarland et al. studied healthy, college-aged subjects without any reported health conditions or gut symptoms and found fully 31 percent had a significant degree of leaky gut. These subjects responded to a trigger meal with a five-fold elevation of blood endotoxin 5 hours later, reflecting both a baseline excess of "bad" gut bacteria, as well as "leakiness" of the gut lining.

Furthermore, blood samples from these subjects showed their innate immune cells *over-reacted* across the board to challenges with other immunogenic substances. This suggests that leaky gut may predispose even healthy young people to inflammation-related diseases and autoimmunity down the line, if not identified and corrected early in life. As we've said, the antecedents of late-life memory loss start as early as 20 years before symptoms appear, and this data suggests that even 20-somethings can benefit from adopting a preventive, brain-healthy diet and lifestyle.

Are All Probiotics Equally Beneficial? Here's One That Stands Out

There *is* a bright side to the leaky gut epidemic. In the same study described above, researchers found that a simple 30-day probiotic treatment reduced levels of post-trigger meal endotoxemia by an average of 42 percent, *without* the subjects even changing their diet or lifestyle. The key is that this was not just *any* probiotic supplement, but a combination of five "spore-forming" bacteria strains (*Bacilli indicus, clausii, subtilis, coagulans,* and *licheniformis*).

Spore-forming bacteria are purported to better survive stomach acid due to their thick protective wall (i.e., the "spore,") and deliver a much higher concentration of "good" bacteria to the small intestine than non-spore probiotics prevalent in the market today. A 42-percent reduction of gut leakiness in just 30 days, without any change in diet, is *highly* significant. The researchers speculate that extending the treatment to 60 days may yield even greater benefits, and further studies are in the works.

While research on spore-forming bacteria is cutting edge, so far, they have proven to be as safe as any other probiotic on the market and are now my first-line choice for probiotic therapy. Interestingly, this study superseded the prevalent clinical precaution of avoiding probiotics in patients with leaky gut, to presumably prevent an increase in endotoxemia by increasing bacterial numbers, even of the "good" kind. It provides evidence that this may not be a concern, rather, that introducing high numbers of beneficial bacteria may help *heal* leaky gut, while *reducing* endo-toxemia markedly.

Restoring beneficial bacteria predicts numerous side-ben-efits beyond healing leaky gut such as better nutrient absorp-tion, more energy and less fatigue and "brain fog" after meals. I'm going to be watching closely to see if products containing the previously mentioned bacteria strains deliver noticeably bet-ter results in clinical practice. So far, the reports back from my patients about their superior benefits are encouraging.

Evaluating Your Gut

If you suffer from conditions such as bloating, flatulence, diarrhea, constipation, or other abdominal symptoms, testing your gut function, leakiness, and your microbiome composition may be particularly useful. Microbiome self-testing is available online, which will tell you how plentiful your beneficial bacteria are, and the quantity of unhealthy strains and yeast. For parasite testing, SIBO testing for small intestinal bacterial overgrowth, zonulin levels, and lactulose/mannitol tests (indicators of leaky gut), food sensitivities, and further gut function evaluation, it may be necessary to visit a functional medicine-trained doctor who can order the tests for you from a specialty lab.

If you live in Australia, "i-screen" at *www.i-screen.com.au* pro-vides comprehensive gut testing comparable to what I can order as a physician here in the U.S. If you are lucky enough to live in Australia, you may wish to avail yourself of this valuable resource that will give you a full-spectrum view of your gut health at an affordable fee. More such "direct-to-consumer" lab tests that you can do without a doctor's prescription are coming on the market online. (Note: An internet search may reveal self-testing available beyond what is mentioned here.)

Ultimately, testing is something to be discussed between you and your doctor. There are several symptoms that are red flag warnings to see your doctor as soon as you can. If you begin to have blood in your stool, start getting cramps, suffer from diarrhea or constipation when you normally don't, or if there are any other major changes to your bowel habits, please seek out your doctor without delay.

Before visiting healers or alternative practitioners, get checked to rule out anything that may need medical attention. I have seen too many patients delay conventional medical evaluation while their condition progressed, and valuable time was wasted. It is wise to consult your doctor to ensure that there is nothing serious that needs medical attention before you attempt self-tests or alternative approaches. The earlier a doctor diagnoses a problem, the easier it is to solve it. When it comes to your gut, waiting too long to address new symptoms can result in serious consequences.

The Ayurveda Approach to Digestion

Burgeoning research on gut health and the microbiome has made it crystal clear that the health of our bodies as a whole depends on the optimal functioning of our digestive tract. Throughout history, Ayurveda has maintained that proper is foundational to good health as well as longevity. It describes that completely digested food turns into "*ojas*," a life-supporting material that keeps the body healthy. Ayurvedic wisdom focuses on correcting digestive imbalances to correct chronic health problems, as well as promoting optimal energy, mood, mental clarity, skin and hair health, and simply feeling your best every day.

While healthy food choices and eating habits are obvious, Ayurveda offers a profound additional perspective on optimizing health by improving your digestion. Rather than giving everyone the same diet and eating recommendations, Ayurveda looks at digestion in terms of three intelligent bodily "software programs," called *doshas*. Depending on one's genetics and dietary and lifestyle habits, imbalances in one or more doshas, accompanied by disturbances in their respective bodily functions, can occur.

The "skinny" on doshas is simple. While modern medicine looks at the body as composed of molecules, cells, tissues, organs, and systems—and has a specialist for each system, GI, neurology, etc., who looks at only *that* part of the body, Ayurveda looks at what is common to *all* the systems. While also acknowledging the heart, circulation, digestive tract, nervous system—Ayurveda knew the functions and role of each of those—it focuses on the common functions of all the systems: movement, metabolism and structure. To be alive, our body needs these three fundamental mega-functions: to circulate and move within and without; to burn fuel for energy, or "metabolize"; and to maintain a structure—skin, bones, muscle, etc.—that holds it all together.

These three "super-systems," as I call them, are each governed or run by their own intelligence, their own "software," programmed in our genes. If we eat, drink, sleep, exercise and otherwise live in a balanced, healthy way, these innate bodily "programs" keep us healthy, youthful and alive for a long time. If we constantly challenge and disrupt bodily functions with irregular sleep, toxic foods and drink, sedentary living, etc., we can eventually override our bodies' inherent ability to "right" itself in response to challenges, and uncomfortable symptoms and outright illness can occur.

Our Genetic Characteristics—
Ayurveda Called Our "Constitution"

A growing body of research is validating Ayurvedic concepts, including that of individual "constitution," an inborn tendency for certain traits that tend to "cluster" into what Ayurveda calls "constitutional type" or "body type." Machine learning and genetic analysis are both yielding support for the three-dosha, or "tridosha" theory of Ayurveda.

Dr. Bredesen himself has written a paper relating the three main subtypes of Alzheimer's disease, with "Inflammatory" due to overly *fiery pitta,* "Atrophic" due to excessively *dry and degenerating vata,* and "Toxic" to *vile,* indirectly related to kapha through imbalanced bacteria, fungi, molds and viruses, accumulation of foreign material, disturbed immune function and other indirect attributes of imbalanced kapha (also known in Ayurveda as "ama").

In my experience, balancing your doshas can be a substantial aid to recovering brain health, and as we saw in Chapter Two, Jeannie found it key to her early recovery, even before she completed her cognoscopy and corrected her nutrient and hormone imbalances. Let's consider how Ayurvedic understanding of the three doshas can help you balance your gut and support your brain and whole-body healing at the same time.

Your Digestive "Type"

When it comes to digestion, you likely have a predominance of one of three main digestive types: airy, fiery, or earthy (*vata, pitta,* or *kapha,*) based on your unique makeup and your lifestyle habits. When in balance, regardless of your type, your digestive system operates smoothly. However, imbalance of any of the three *doshas* results in characteristic signs and symptoms—often long before actual disease develops—which are usually correctable through specific dietary, herbal, and lifestyle approaches. Let's take a closer look at the three supersystems that Ayurveda tells us "run the show" in our bodies every day.

Vata, the "airy" supersystem, governs all movement of the body; it guides secretion of hormones, circulation, and communication through the nervous system—including the pivotal vagus nerve. *Vata* controls movement through the digestive tract and

74

the whole body; it is the *dosha* of movement. An imbalance of *vata* can express as reflux (reverse movement) or constipation (inhibited movement). It may also manifest as excess air.

Classic symptoms of *vata* imbalance include gas, excess belching, flatulence, or bloating—each having to do with the air element. *Vata* imbalance also brings variability, such as unpredictable hunger, fluctuating appetite, and a tendency towards irritable bowel—meaning the stool changes often between loose, soft, hard and constipated.

Pitta is in charge of transformation, digestion, and metabolism. Dealing with acids and enzymes, *pitta* breaks down food from complex to simple molecules for digestion. *Pitta* is a fiery element, with its heat expressing physically as heartburn, burning sensations, or sour or acidic stomach.

An imbalanced *pitta* results in feeling heartburn, burning sensations, overly hungry or feeling irritable, angry, or "hot-tempered" when food is delayed, or a meal skipped. There is a tendency for frequent soft or loose stools as the heat "melts" fat and waste, typically leading to softer stool.

Kapha is responsible for bodily strength, structure, and mucus linings. It supports the integrity of the intestinal lining and the tight junctions to help prevent increased intestinal permeability.

When there is imbalance of *kapha* in the gut, one can feel heavy or sleepy after eating, food feels like it "just sits" in the stomach, often for hours, and it takes many hours to become hungry again, which is even then rarely intense. Stools can be sticky or have noticeable mucus.

Fortunately, each of the three types of digestive imbalances is correctable through remedies of foods, spices, herbs, and eating habits specific to the type of *dosha*. I recommend you take the quiz at *www.drnancyhealth.com* (described below) to find out your type and get personalized tips to help you restore and keep your digestion in top operating form.

Spice Up Your Digestive System

The allure of spices is much more than just flavor to a meal. Thousands of research articles verify the healing power of spices, and their ability to support digestion while reducing inflammation. In a study done at the International Laboratory for Advanced Biomedicine, researchers demonstrated that spice-derived compounds interact with multiple biochemical targets and help counter imbalanced inflammatory pathways and factors associated with chronic diseases. They found a wide range of benefits from spices that are present in nearly every pantry worldwide. Below are a few examples:

Spice	Benefits for Digestion
Black Pepper	The piperine in black pepper eases digestion and stimulates hydrochloric acid production by the stomach, promoting better digestion of proteins in food. It also supports absorption, including of brain-saving curcumin from the "superstar spice," turmeric.
Fennel	Relaxes the smooth muscles of the gastrointestinal system which helps reduce gas, bloating, and stomach cramps. Shown to be useful in easing colic in babies.
Cumin	Increases the activity of digestive enzymes, potentially speeding up digestion. Promotes release of bile from the liver which helps digestion of fats and certain nutrients in the gut.
Coriander	Helps with upset stomach, loss of appetite, nausea, diarrhea, bowel spasms, and intestinal gas. Also stimulates enzymatic activity in the liver, including detox enzymes.

Spice	Benefits for Digestion
Ginger	Helps relieve IBS symptoms, gas, nausea, and heartburn. (However, avoid if stomach burning is a predominant symptom, as ginger is itself a bit heating.) Boosts nutrient absorption and supports growth of beneficial bacteria.
Rosemary	Stimulates appetite and improves gastric tone, allowing food to be more easily digested.
Mint	Increases bile secretion and encourages bile flow, which helps to speed and ease digestion, especially of fats. Also supports mental alertness and productivity, potentially helpful to counter sleepiness after eating.
Turmeric	Supports digestion by relaxing the smooth muscles on the walls of the intestines and gently pushing food through the intestines. Promotes bile flow and helps prevent gas and bloating as food is being digested. Supports detox processes in the liver. Antioxidant and powerfully anti-inflammatory, turmeric has been found to directly inhibit amyloid formation in the brain.

Optimizing Your Unique Digestive System

You may be thinking "I don't have any digestive symptoms; my digestion seems to be good." Great! Maybe you are doing just fine. On the other hand, as we saw in the leaky gut study quoted earlier, you don't have to have digestive symptoms to have leaky gut, excess inflammation, or a digestion-related disorder. There are a wide variety of ailments caused or influenced by the gut that do not manifest directly in the digestive system.

If you have any of the chronic symptoms already mentioned, or simply want to feel better physically or mentally, take the Digestive Quiz. Finding out your specific digestive type and implementing personalized advice to your digestive type will help you improve your overall health.

Take the Digestive Quiz

Check out the digestive quiz at *www.drnancyhealth.com* to determine your Ayurvedic digestive type. You'll receive personalized tips for your type, once a week for six weeks, to help optimize and balance your but health a la Ayurveda. Often, taking those simple measures can be enough to restore good digestion, resolve functional symptoms and improve your energy and vitality. With just one tip a week, it's easy to integrate and usually bestows benefits beyond those available through Western medicine, Western herbology and Functional Medicine approaches.

Beverly's Story—IBS Solved

Beverly is a 52-year-old radio host with a show on health who came to me with a diagnosis of irritable bowel syndrome (IBS). She related that she had suffered from intestinal cramps, gas, bloating, and loose stools almost every day after lunch for years. Her doctor had diagnosed IBS, or "irritable bowel syndrome," and prescribed a drug that didn't help her, and she preferred to forego in favor of natural approaches anyway.

All the supplements she had tried—and there were many—had not done the trick and she was getting frustrated that with all her knowledge of natural health, she couldn't resolve her condition. She shared with me, "I eat so healthy. I just don't understand why I have this problem."

When I went more deeply into her health history and her diet, I saw clearly that her diet was, in fact, healthy by everyday standards. She was eating vegetables and salads for lunch every day. It was all wholesome, natural, and non-processed; however, most of the vegetables she ate were raw.

However, with her cramps, gas, and thin body type, I knew raw foods could easily trigger irregularity in her bowels, which are governed by the movement super-system, *vata*. Raw, rough, coarse, and cold all aggravate the nerves that govern peristalsis and that could be what was triggering her bowel movement into such irregular and uncomfortable actions.

What we call "vata-balancing" measures were in order. I recommended first that Beverly replace her ice water with hot water, especially around mealtimes, to promote smooth peristalsis. (Interestingly, one of my clinical practice journals reported that hot water is an effective and instantaneous cure for esophageal spasm, evidencing its value in promoting smooth downward flow through the gut.) According to Ayurveda, hot water also increases digestive strength—sense-making, since digestion is chemistry, which always takes place faster and more thoroughly in warm temperatures.

Next, I recommended she replace her raw vegetables and salads with cooked vegetables for lunch, along with plenty of healthy oils and ideally some soothing digestive spices such as cumin and fennel.

Two months later, Beverly wrote to say that her irritable bowel syndrome had dissipated within days of changing her diet. On follow-up two years later, she confirmed that her IBS had never come back. She was eating cooked meals at lunchtime, felt fantastic, and was very grateful.

Cooked or Raw—Which Is Better?

If there's one thing my 30-plus years of clinical experience has taught, it's that "everyone's different." What works for one may not work for another. While Ayurveda favors cooked food, spiced, and eaten at proper times for optimal digestion and absorption, I have patients who have been helped by raw diets as well—for a time.

The most common story I hear from patients who "went raw," is that they no longer are—at least, not completely. The usual report is they got great results in the first few months, often resolving a variety of chronic ills. After some time, however, they started to feel less well on the all-raw routine, and eventually re-introduced cooked food, at least in part, usually without losing any of the health benefits they originally gained from their raw food months.

Why is this so common? I've observed that rigid adherence to any diet or path of lifestyle, without regard to the feedback of the body over time, often "backfires" in nutritional deficiencies and lack of vigor and vitality, if not frank symptoms. Anything too extreme usually ends up creating some imbalance over time and needs to be adjusted. In general, steer clear of rigid dogma, listen to your body and adjust your behavior accordingly. Some raw vegetables and fruits are great to include in your daily diet, if you digest them well, without symptoms. Your body and your taste buds will guide you in choosing the right proportion of raw vs. cooked for you. Keep in mind that "balance" is a dynamic state, and what is right for you may change day by day, season-to season, after travel, trauma or surgery, according to age, or from other factors. Your body's own inner intelligence is the "ultimate Ayurveda."

Care in Cooking: To Boil, To Microwave, To Bust

Research on raw versus cooked vegetables reveals that some lose antioxidants and nutrients with cooking, and some actually *gain* nutrient value, not to mention bioavailability. For example, it is well documented that lycopene is more bioavailable from cooked tomatoes than from raw. Carrots, celery, and green beans all *increased* in antioxidant power from cooking, to name just a few examples.

One of the caveats of cooking is how to do it to maximize nutrient retention. Papers conflict regarding which cooking methods retain the most nutrients—steaming, boiling, grilling, microwaving, pressure-cooking, baking, and frying—at least in part due to which vegetables and which constituents or properties are being measured. Boiling generally loses across the board, with many nutrients leaching into the water. (In theory, you can reclaim the nutrients by drinking the water with your meal, though be careful about the pot material, which may diffuse into the water with prolonged boiling.)

Jimenez-Monreal et al. conclude that cooking methods with least water are preferable, declaring "water is not the cook's best friend when it comes to preparing vegetables," and I might add, not the diner's best friend either due to loss of nutrient value!

Another important point about cooking methods has to do with microwaving.

In a measure of antioxidant activity, critical to curbing the collateral damage of inflammation, a study in the *Journal of the Science of Food and Agriculture,* found that broccoli lost 75 to 90 percent of its key antioxidant compounds after microwaving, whereas steaming *preserved* 89 to 100 percent of them.

While study results do vary, intuitively, my "Ayurvedic" take on microwaving is that the very high energy agitation and irregular heating of the food imparts a quality of subtle imbalance (i.e., in *vata,* the movement principle, primarily) that may influence the same *dosha* in the eater. Clinically, this seems to have been the case in a few select examples in my practice across the years.

As this may sound a bit esoteric or far-fetched (even to me!), I felt my intuition was validated by an article published on the topic in, of all places, a *physics* journal. Eke et al., in the *Journal of Radiation Research and Applied Sciences,* reported in 2017 that microwaved food fed to rats, as compared to unmicrowaved, resulted in a lowering of the animals' endogenous antioxidant enzyme activity as well as levels of two leading antioxidant vitamins, A and E. The fact that the effect was "dose-dependent," meaning longer microwaving times was associated with more detrimental effect, added further support for the validity of the findings.

Furthermore, the scientists provided a graphic "inner look" at the effect of microwaving on food molecules that struck a chord with my Ayurvedic instincts. After citing multiple studies on how microwaved food can adversely affect blood cells, increase inflammatory cells, change heart rate and contain carcinogens, the authors speculated that microwaving may have a deleterious effect on the health-giving properties of food.

Citing multiple references as they write, Eke et al. eloquently expound, in a microscopically accurate and graphic manner only a physicist would be capable of, that "the alternating microwave electric current generated by the magnetron in every microwave oven, forces the food molecules to rotate at the frequency of 1 to 100 billion times per second. The friction from this violent, thrashing motion tears at the food, vitamin and enzyme molecules, destroying, for instance, their cells' walls, while heating them savagely and changing their shape." Sounds like a recipe for an Ayurvedic "movement" or *vata* imbalance, if ever I heard one! I hope it's enough to inspire you to pack up the microwave, just as I did over twenty years ago.

Tips for Every Digestive Type

Whether you are suffering from bloating, heartburn, or are just looking to boost your digestive system, here are a few tips for a healthy gut from ancient Ayurveda that are just as relevant today.

- Eat fresh, organic, non-genetically engineered food. It is preferable to eat organic food to avoid consuming toxins in the form of synthetic herbicides and pesticides. For example, the ubiquitous herbicide glyphosate (found in Roundup®) is showing up in many non-organic foods these days, and besides increasing cancer risk, has been shown to disrupt gut bacteria and gut lining integrity. Avoid it!

- Avoid unhealthy fats such as the trans fats found in dough-nuts, French fries, and any foods that are fried in a high heat.
- Do not consume curdled products at night. The sticki-ness of curds, including yogurt, kefir, and cheeses (dairy or non-dairy) can be difficult for our bodies to digest and when consumed in the evening lead to blockage according to Ayurveda. Notice if morning congestion and joint stiff-ness improve by following this rule for dinner. Also, nuts in the evening can stress the gut and potentially even promote blockage.
- Include spices and herbs in your cooking. As we've seen, spices are potent suppliers of antioxidants that can boost your immune system and reduce inflammation.
- Avoid leftovers or stale and heavily processed food. For example, when the starches in wheat and potatoes are cooked and then refrigerated, it turns into what is called retrograde starch, and becomes difficult to digest. These foods are likely to give you gas, bloating, and disturb the gut health. While it is trendy today to recommend cooking and cooling grains in order to *promote* retrograde starch to reduce carbohydrate load, it is not recommended Ayurvedically, as it promotes *ama*, or undigested food molecules, a direct contributor to leaky gut (which Ayurveda described over 5,000 years ago).
- Eat the largest and heaviest meal of the day at lunchtime, before 2 p.m., when your digestive strength is at its strongest.
- Do not overeat. Leave at least one-third of your stomach vol-ume for the digestion process.
- Avoid cold or iced water before, during, and after a meal, as it inhibits the digestion process. If you're thirsty, sip small amounts of warm water with the meal. Warm water with a squeeze of lemon or lime is tasty and at the same time, helps

the body extract minerals from the food and supports over-all digestion.

- Always sit down when you eat or drink.
- Avoid stimulation during meals such as eating at your desk, reading, working on the computer, watching television, talking on the phone, or engaging in emotional conversations. Focus on what's going into your body to avoid over-eating and to promote good digestion. Remember, digestion is governed by our parasympathetic nervous system, the "rest and digest" one.
- Enhance your digestion by taking it easy for about five minutes after you've finished eating, before you get up and resume your day.
- Take enough time between meals to fully digest one meal before starting the next.
- Include probiotics and prebiotics. Probiotics can be found in dairy and non-dairy forms of yogurt, kefir, and in other fermented foods. Prebiotics are a special form of dietary fiber that acts as a fertilizer for the good bacteria in your gut, particularly in the lower intestine. Prebiotics are found in a number of specialized food sources as well as asparagus, Jerusalem artichoke and dandelion greens. Consult your doctor about whether a probiotic supplement or spore-forming probiotic may be appropriate for you.

Take This Simple Action #3 Now!

Balance your diet according to your digestive type and you'll accomplish the first step towards optimal gut health.

Go to *www.thehealthybrainsolution.com/gut* and take the short quiz to discover your type and get one highly doable "tip for your type" each week for the next 6 weeks.

www.thehealthybrainsolution.com/gut

4

Conquer Your Carbs to Boost Brain Power

Is Alzheimer's Disease "Type 3 Diabetes"?

—Suzanne de la Monte, MD, PhD

Key #4: Optimize Your Blood Sugar

To the question, "Is Alzheimer's Disease 'Type 3 Diabetes'?" Suzanne de la Monte and colleagues provide an emphatic "yes." One of the first to recognize the foundational role of insulin resistance in Alzheimer's pathology, Dr. de la Monte puts it aptly, "Whether primary or secondary in origin, insulin resistance initiates a cascade of neurodegeneration that is propagated by metabolic dysfunction, increased oxidative stress, neuro-inflammation, impaired cell survival, and disturbed lipid metabolism. These injurious processes compromise neuronal and glial functions. ..."

To put it simply, insulin resistance is front and center of a complicated network of interrelated metabolic functions gone awry, all culminating in increased amyloid (and tau) deposition. To make matters worse, amyloid in turn feeds back to fuel the same factors that triggered it.

This vicious cycle of disturbed sugar metabolism affects such diverse body regions as the gut, circulatory channels, immune system, brain tissue, repair (glial cells), nerve cells, and cellular components, "cell organelles," including those responsible for energy production (mitochondria), lipid synthesis (endoplasmic reticulum), and other critical cellular functions.

Dr. de la Monte and her colleagues are prominent pioneers, among the first to call for a multifaceted approach to researching, preventing, and treating Alzheimer's, rather than the usual, narrow, "pill for an ill" approach. Rather, their work has helped establish Alzheimer's as a heterogeneous condition with a multitude of causes, including disturbed carbohydrate metabolism.

Let's take a look at the role sugar metabolism plays in health and how it creates disease when it goes awry. ...

Just What *Is* Sugar and What Does the Body Do With It?

Sugar is essentially a simple 1- to 2-molecule carbohydrate that our body either burns as energy or converts to fat. There are a few main forms of the simplest sugar molecules, including glucose, sucrose, galactose, and fructose. Digestion of sugar and more complex carbohydrates requires a series of biochemical actions that start in the mouth with the salivary enzyme called "amylase" and continues in the stomach.

Once the broken-down carbohydrates pass from the stomach into the intestines, the pancreas releases enzymes that complete the digestive process. Simple carbohydrates that have been broken down into glucose (the end-product of carbohydrate digestion) pass through the intestinal lining and straight into the bloodstream.

Key point: As soon as your body detects sugar in the blood, your pancreas releases insulin to drive the sugar into your cells to be used for fuel. Any leftover glucose is sent to your liver or muscles to be stored as glycogen, where it can be accessed when the body needs a rush of energy. When more simple carbs flood the body than it needs or can store as glycogen, the carbs are stored as fat. (Just an aside—isn't that amazing? Sugar is converted into fat—but somehow we, as women, knew that!)

What is Insulin Resistance?

Insulin resistance develops when the body loses its ability to respond properly to the insulin made by the pancreas. The more sugar we ingest, the more glucose pours into the bloodstream, and the more insulin the pancreas makes in response. Eventually, our cells call out "no more sugar!" and stop absorbing it from the blood. They "just say no" to our insulin, "resisting" its usual effects.

In response, the pancreas strains to make more and more of the very hormone the body is rejecting. All the while, cells continue to resist its message to absorb glucose from the blood and blood glucose levels rise. Diabetes is setting in, and type 1.5 Alzheimer's, "diabetes of the brain" is following close behind.

Such "insulin resistance" is the *sine qua non* of diabetes. Currently, over 9 percent of Americans have been diagnosed with diabetes. Moreover, in 2015, research by the Alameda Health System in California, found that nearly one in every three adults in the U.S., over 100 million people, and half of those aged 60 years and older, had some degree of insulin resistance, a "pre-diabetic" condition.

Cognitive symptoms of insulin resistance, or early "diabetes of the brain," can manifest as lethargy, mental fatigue, excess hunger, forgetfulness and brain fog. If not corrected, ideally through diet and exercise, or controlled through medication, chronic insulin resistance is a major risk factor for dementia down the line.

Insulin resistance commonly coexists in people who are

- Obese or overweight
- Consuming a high sugar or high carb diet
- Living a sedentary lifestyle
- Suffering from chronic stress
- Suffering from a hormonal imbalance from conditions such as PCOS (polycystic ovary syndrome,)

or

- Have high levels of inflammation.
- Have non-alcoholic steatohepatitis (NASH; "fatty liver").

Don't We Need Sugar?

Our bodies require glucose to create the energy that keeps us moving. However, we don't have to *eat* sugar to get it—and had better not. Our bodies were designed to create all the blood sugar, "glucose," that we need from complex carbohydrates, fats, and proteins naturally found in the whole foods Nature provides. Extracting sugar and other sweeteners from foods, concentrating them, and adding them to yet other, more processed foods, to make them more appealing (read "boost sales and consumption") are modern phenomena that our bodies were not designed to handle.

Keep in mind that added sugars are generally overly refined, have no nutritional value beyond the calories, and contain no protein, vitamins, or minerals for your body. Moreover, the dangers of sugar go far beyond its "empty calories."

Excess sugar is literally toxic to brain cells. Conversely, an optimal level of blood sugar—not too high—has been cited as perhaps *the* most important factor in preventing Alzheimer's and in healing the brain from cognitive decline.

Imbalanced sugar metabolism harms our brains in two ways. First of all, sugar directly damages neurons and promotes amyloid formation. Secondly, when nerve cells become "resistant" to insulin, they also become resistant to the supportive, healing effects of insulin, which is also a potent neuronal growth factor - a double deprivation.

Moreover, research shows that excess sugar ingestion and elevated blood glucose lead to *inflammation*, potentially damaging to all bodily tissues and organs, particularly the liver and pancreas, which overwork in attempt to combat the overload of glucose from excessive dietary sugar and carbohydrate ingestion.

If sugar is so bad, why do so many of us crave it? We crave sweetness for a simple evolutionary reason; sweet tasting food, which was historically wholesome, "whole food," rich in nutrients, was difficult to come by. It promoted quick energy and rapid weight gain, a protective buffer for the "in-between" times when food was scarce. Yet in our modern times with overabundant, constant food sources, indulging in refined sweets is anything but an evolutionary advantage.

The Sweet Poison: Are You Addicted?

While "addiction" is a strong word, wellness expert Dr. Alan Greene, who authored several children's health books, warns consumers that there is mounting evidence that too much sugar can lead to genuine biochemical addiction.

When we consume sugar, particularly refined or processed sugar, our brain releases dopamine—a neurotransmitter that tells the brain that what it just experienced is worth getting more of. Dopamine is our brain neurotransmitter in charge of reward and reinforcement. As children, we finished our vegetables and received dessert as a reward—a double behavioral and biochemical learning. When our brain receives dopamine from the sweet reward, it begins to program us to want more.

Other substances that release dopamine include nicotine, heroin, and cocaine. They all stimulate dopamine release, which fuels the "high" that users experience. When the dopamine wears off; users are left seeking another boost. Research done on laboratory rats found that Oreo™ cookies activated more neurons in the brain's pleasure centers than cocaine does, creating addiction motivated by sugar's sweet rewards.

While it can be dramatic to call sugar a poison, the damaging effects overconsumption can have on our bodies deservedly earn sugar the title "toxic substance." On the other hand, fruits, vegetables, grains, and other whole food sources of carbohydrates (which are composed of sugars bound together,) provide a ready and safe, "slow infusion" of blood glucose to fuel our metabolism.

In summary, carbohydrates we consume are broken down into glucose before being absorbed into the blood, stimulating insulin release which drives glucose into our cells for immediate energy or short-term storage as glycogen. These processes are kept in balance by our "sugar-handling system," including insulin and other hormones as well as enzymes in our liver, muscle, and other cells.

While the body has this built-in system for metabolizing carbs and sugar, the problem is that most Americans currently consume more refined, processed sugar than the system was designed to handle. Various forms of sugar are added to most processed and packaged foods to "enhance" flavor, fuel addiction and encourage repeat consumption, at the price of powering the modern-day epidemic of insulin resistance, diabetes and dementia growing in our nation, and worldwide.

Americans indeed consume an inordinate amount of refined sugar daily, an average of 30 teaspoons, or a full hundred pounds of sugar per person, per year. Yet our bodies are only designed to handle one-tenth of that, a maximum of 3 teaspoons per day. For example, just one can of cola with its 8 teaspoons of sugar effectively overdoses our sugar-handling capacity by two and one-half times! So, check your recipes and product labels for their sugar content: 1 tsp. $\cong$ 5 grams. Keep your daily intake at 15 grams or below (not an easy feat if you eat packaged foods).

Keep in mind that added sugars are generally overly refined, have no nutritional value beyond simple calories, and contain no protein, vitamins, or minerals for your body. And, as we saw above, the dangers of sugar go beyond its feature of "empty calories.

The Sugar Scandal

Try as we might as individuals to eat right and stay healthy, we are as a nation at the mercy of the media, and of market forces that shape the outcomes of even "objective, scientific" research and its reporting. Recall the 1960s: butter is bad, margarine is good. Then the 2000s, margarine is bad, butter is better. 1960s: Sugar is fine, fat is bad. 2010s: Fat is great, sugar is the enemy. Confused? Cynical? You have every right to be. Yet finally, after 50 years, the light of truth is starting to shine as decades of data create clarity in the heretofore murky field of nutrition and health.

One of the greatest health deceptions of all time revolves around sugar and ended up needlessly costing millions of Americans their lives. In the 1960s, the United States scrambled to take control of the heart disease epidemic that was steadily on the rise. While the concept that what we ate could affect our heart was relatively new in Western medicine, evidence was mounting that refined sugar consumption was an important risk factor. After former President Eisenhower suffered from a cardiac episode, scientists were put to task to discover the causes of heart disease and what could be done to prevent it.

In 2016, compelling evidence was uncovered and published in *JAMA Internal Medicine*, that the Sugar Research Foundation had secretly funded scientists in 1967 to publish a guileful review article in *The New England Journal of Medicine* discounting accumulating data that sugar consumption was a major factor in coronary heart disease, and aiming a diversionary, "ivory tower" finger at dietary fat instead.

Despite growing evidence that a high-sugar diet led to conditions such as diabetes, cancer, and other long-term illnesses, the sugar industry reportedly lent financial support behind the scenes to steer the conclusions of the study away from sugar as a potential problem. Instead, the research review stated there were major problems with all studies that implicated sugar and, concluded that cutting fat out of American diets was the way to prevent heart disease.

These "findings," funded by the Sugar Research Foundation, set the nation on a low-fat frenzy that lasted over 40 years, well into the new millennium. Foods traditionally considered healthy, such as yogurt, were altered to remove the "bad" fat, rendering them less satisfying, which was countered, of course, by adding sugar, securing sugar's role in the western diet, and the growing prosperity of the sugar industry.

It has taken nearly 50 years to correctly rewrite history, and for our country to learn and accept that refined sugars are toxic and healthy, wholesome fats are actually good for us.

Toxins and Your Blood Sugar

While medical authorities are quick to point the finger at our sedentary habits and love affair with sugary foods as the cause of the ever-rising numbers worldwide of insulin-resistance, metabolic syndrome, and diabetes, researchers have uncovered yet another, less obvious, factor that has risen dramatically over the past decades, and is purported to play an equally sinister role—environmental toxins.

Substances as diverse as nitrosamines in our food, agricultural nitrates in our water, pesticides, herbicides, plastics, and likely many other man-made substances are now implicated as major disruptors of our endocrine systems, triggering disturbed metabolism, insulin resistance, obesity, polycystic ovary syndrome, NASH, and neurodegenerative diseases including Parkinson's and Alzheimer's.

Researchers have discovered that one particular enzyme, glucokinase, which helps signal how much insulin the pancreas should produce at a given blood sugar level, appears to be "defunct" in those with a type of pre-diabetes characterized by a high fasting glucose level. Based on her study, researcher Leigh

Perreault at the University of Colorado School of Medicine in Denver observes that the condition occurs even in "healthy" people of normal weight with no reason to have insulin resistance. Only a tiny fraction of those with the condition are genetically predisposed, nor are they older or more overweight than normal subjects.

For most, "we think the problem lies somewhere else," Perreault says. "We think maybe they are exposed to some kind of environmental pollutant that interferes with glucokinase." The possibilities are vast, "everything from saturated fats to plasticizers to pesticides," she says. "We're screening all the weird, icky junk that's out there."

Perreault's work is just one sampling in a burgeoning field of research into EDCs (endocrine-disrupting chemicals) and our health, including cognitive health. Sakkiah et al. reported recently on the ability of EDCs to disrupt our hormonal functions, including insulin and blood sugar regulation, by binding to and stimulating receptors that normally are meant for our body's own natural hormones. Disturbed signaling at these receptors is associated with increased incidence of diabetes, obesity, breast, and prostate cancer, infertility, stroke, and, not least, Alzheimer's.

We'll delve further into toxic causes of cognitive decline and how to correct them in Chapter Seven. Meanwhile, let's circle back to what we can do to stem the tide of sugar overload in our lives and protect our bodies and brains from insulin resistance and its related risks.

We Can't Get Away With What We Used To

While aging does not automatically preordain insulin resistance, as our body ages it does change. Body fat and fat cell size increase with age and our muscles—major players in insulin sensitivity—begin to weaken and shrink. In award-winning research, Dr. Orville Kolterman and his team concluded that along with increasing body fat and dwindling muscle mass, our bodies become less able to process refined sugars with age. His group verified that this inability to use our insulin can lead to a long list of complications, including inflammation, diabetes, and Alzheimer's disease.

Menopause: A Risk To Metabolism and Our Brains

For women, transitioning into menopause creates an extra concern. Since our body's hormonal systems are interdependent, shifts in our reproductive hormones can trigger changes in other hormone systems, and insulin resistance more readily develops. Cardiovascular disease, insulin resistance, and metabolic syndrome all become more frequent after menopause, as the protective effects of estrogen diminish and underlying metabolic weaknesses can manifest.

Yet we have to remember that there's a lot we can do to mitigate this downward trend. Menopause is a great time to kick the sugar habit and adopt a wholesome diet, if you haven't already. In my clinical experience, going off sugar "cold turkey" usually works best. Cravings usually disappear within a week and stay away as long as you don't eat sugar again. Eating regular meals, with abundant cooked organic vegetables at lunch and dinner, with a protein of your choice and whole carbs, such as quinoa, can be very liberating, and result in spontaneous weight loss without trying. Such effortless weight loss, up to 25 pounds, has occurred over and over in my patients. I highly recommend adopting this sustainable, satisfying approach to "diet," rather than restricting calories or manipulating food groups according to the latest fad.

Ever notice that extra belly fat that nearly every menopausal woman accumulates to some degree? A bit of extra abdominal fat can act as an "estrogen factory" that helps us transition through menopause, since abdominal fat produces more estrogen than fat elsewhere in the body. However, a gain of more than 3 to 5 pounds may promote hormonal imbalance, along with inflammation and insulin resistance, both set-ups for brain degeneration, as well as cardiovascular disease.

Imbalance in our hormones after menopause can also affect how our brain conducts autophagy, reducing the cleaning of toxic or waste matter while we sleep, another potential reason our risk of Alzheimer's and other neurodegenerative illnesses goes up after the "change." Maintaining an eating schedule that optimizes autophagy (explained below), ideally coupled with an early, "Ayurvedic" bedtime can help us get the most rejuvenative sleep and maximize our brain power, even after menopause. (See Chapter Six for more on hormones, sleep, and our brains.)

Sugar Consumption and Your Health

As we've seen, excess sugar consumption, overeating, refined carbohydrates, and packaged foods all contribute to insulin resistance, rising blood sugar levels, obesity, NASH, metabolic syndrome, diabetes, and, of course, Alzheimer's and other neurodegenerative disease. Additional illnesses caused or aggravated by an over-consumption of refined carbohydrates and sugars include:

- gum disease
- heart disease
- attention deficit disorder
- depression
- insomnia
- cancer
- faster aging processes

Kelly's Story: The Ill-Fated Ice Cream Cone

Kelly, a 69-year-old retired schoolteacher, had been diagnosed with mild cognitive impairment a year before I saw her as a patient in my Healthy Brain™ Consultation and Health Coaching Program. I was struck by her story of how dramatically sugar intake affected her cognition, a substance she had learned to strictly avoid. The summer before, however, while car touring with her family across the scorching desert Southwest, her grandkids excitedly begged for an "ice cream stop." Kelly related how, though she knew it wasn't good for her memory, she just couldn't resist having an ice cream cone along with everyone else. In recalling the event, her husband rolled his eyes and they both laughed nervously over how impaired she became within an hour or two. "For 3 to 4 days, she couldn't remember anything—even where we were or where we were going. We had to help her with everything. She really deteriorates when she eats sugar."

Boosting Your Carb Metabolism To Heal Your Brain

As we've seen in previous chapters, Ayurveda has held for millennia that whole body healing begins with "gut health." Through balancing "agni," our processes of digestion and metabolism, and optimizing the food we put into our bodies, we set the conditions for the entire physiology to re-establish balance and good health.

Let's dive deeper into the process of metabolism and what happens when we eat and when we fast. (*Note:* In the course of this chapter, the term "carbs" includes refined sugars as well as any foods our bodies readily convert into glucose, such as fruit, bread, rice, grains, and starchy vegetables.)

As we've seen, when you consume carbs and sugar, your blood sugar rises, and your body secretes insulin to drive the glucose into the cells, where your body will try to burn it for energy. However, when there's no glucose coming down the pike, and we need energy, the body will first draw on stores of glycogen, a stored form of readily available sugar, and when that's depleted, will break down proteins or fat. Fat and protein require extra steps to convert them to energy, so they are "burned" more slowly than sugar.

In the slower process of breaking down fat for fuel, break-down products called "ketones" are formed which the body is able to burn for fuel. In a sense, you can liken our bodies to hybrid cars. We can burn either glucose, a "dirty fuel" like gasoline, that requires oxygen and generates free radicals, or we can burn "clean fuel," ketones.

In fact, burning ketones is so "clean" that the body's house-cleaning mechanisms or autophagy processes get strongly activated during "ketosis" enabling the brain to clean out harmful plaque, including the beta-amyloid of Alzheimer's disease. No wonder that optimizing your blood sugar is one of the seven "keys" to staying sharp after 40, and one of the most powerful at that.

Is Low Glycemic for YOU?

As you begin to select your carbs more consciously, it will be good to keep in mind recent breakthrough research from the Weitzmann Institute in Tel Aviv. You may have noticed it's common today to label foods "high glycemic" or "low glycemic," as if the glycemic index resides in the food itself. However, this fascinating and paradigm-shifting research establishes that different people's blood sugar responses to the same food can vary widely.

Researchers found that each person's body processes carbs and sugar differently, and it can run against common wisdom. For example, while some subjects kept their blood sugar low after a banana and spiked it with a cookie as we'd expect, the blood sugar of some subjects stayed low after the cookie and soared following the banana! How could this be?

Researchers profiled 800 subjects in detail as to their blood parameters, height, weight, waist size, blood pressure, the composition of their gut microbiome, and dietary intake. A cell phone app monitored physical activity and sleep patterns. The researchers were able to develop a formula using machine learning that predicted what foods would be most optimal, glycemically speaking, for any individual. Further tests of this algorithm to guide dietary choices for each person confirmed its usefulness for lowering glycemic responses and improving gut bacterial balance in subjects who followed their highly personalized program.

"One size certainly does not fit all" in the area of diet and glycemic control. That's why monitoring your own glucose and ketones for a few weeks is recommended as part of optimizing your cognition. Measuring your levels gives you a "hack" into your own glucose handling system and helps ensure your diet is one that will keep your metabolism fit and your brain smart through the decades to come.

Please note: If your fasting blood sugar, HgA1c (indicating your average blood sugar over 2 to 3 months) and fasting insulin are optimal, and your weight is low normal or underweight, I *don't* recommend you limit your carbs beyond your usual intake unless you are under a doctor's supervision. Otherwise, you run the risks of getting undernourished and losing excess weight, which can lead to worsening of cognitive decline, and a detrimental effect on your mood and overall level of functioning.

The "Ketoflex 12/3" Intermittent Fast for Brain Healing

In his therapeutic approach, Dr. Bredesen suggests what he refers to as the "Ketoflex 12/3" program to help lower blood sugar and support the brain's nightly internal cleansing, As we've seen, both blood sugar control and "autophagy," the brain's internal housekeeping mechanism, are key processes that quell neurodegeneration and insulin resistance.

In Ketoflex 12/3, one avoids eating for at least 3 hours before bed, and fasts for at least 12 full hours from dinner to breakfast.

This timing allows the body to "flex" between burning glucose during the day, and shifting into burning ketones, "ketosis" during the night. This recommended timing echoes Ayurvedic theory, which states that the period between 10 p.m. to 2 a.m. is a time when the body is getting rid of toxins, or ama, metabolizing wastes, and rejuvenating the body.

Ketoflex 12/3 is essentially a ketogenic diet, which encourages our metabolism to shift to burning fats instead of glucose, for at least several hours during the day, as well as through the night. To achieve this, Ketoflex 12/3 recommends that you fast for a minimum period of 12 hours, from night to morning and avoid eating three hours before going to sleep, as well as following a wholesome diet, avoiding sugar and refined carbs.

Recent research has found that such "intermittent fasting" such as the Ketoflex 12/3 program, in which eating is restricted to a limited period in each 24-hour daily cycle, helps improve glucose intolerance, reduce memory loss, and regulate hormone metabolism. It's definitely a practice I believe just about everyone should begin to follow right away, (with the exception of those who are underweight or undernourished, as described above.) Simply make it part of your ongoing preventive lifestyle, whether your testing shows that your sugar-handling is compromised, or not.

I've had numerous patients tell me that their healthy habits such as this and bringing home-cooked organic vegetable meals to work, have even inspired their co-workers, friends, and colleagues to adopt healthier habits themselves. You may just help others save their lives and health too!

Meanwhile, fasting for 12 hours from dinner to breakfast can be difficult in the beginning, especially if you are already suffering from insulin resistance. If you find you're especially hungry in the early days of following Ketoflex 12/3, you can take one-half to

1 teaspoon of MCT oil (medium chain triglycerides), which helps the brain and body shift into the ketone-burning mode (ketosis).

Taking 1 teaspoon of MCT oil one to three times daily, increasing gradually as needed to a maximum of 1 tablespoon three times daily, can help mitigate hunger and promote the flexible transitioning of the body between glucose-burning and ketone-burning states. Alternatively, you may take organic coconut oil in the same amounts, if you prefer a "whole food" source of MCTs.

If you have the ApoE4 gene type, your body may be more sensitive to the potentially deleterious effects of sustained intake of saturated fats such as MCT oil, coconut oil, and ghee (clarified butter, Ayurveda's preferred oil for the brain, and a rich source of MCTs). Therefore, after you have used these oils for a few weeks and have become more metabolically "flexible"; i.e., can smoothly switch between glucose- and ketone-burning states as evidenced by comfortably fasting for 12 to 14 hours without excessive hunger or weakness, it's advisable to substitute organic olive or avocado oil for the saturated, MCT-rich oils in your diet.

Another "hunger-buster," especially if it's "false hunger," is to drink some plain hot water, hot water with lemon, or an herbal tea when hunger pangs strike between your designated mealtimes. According to Ayurveda, this practice helps "burn off" and flush out ama, or wastes, being digested during our fasting hours. This description parallels the modern understanding that fasting does in fact promote an internal "housecleaning" mode, (scientifically termed "autophagy,") another validation of an ancient Ayurvedic concept that we can take advantage of for a sharper brain today.

Why Not to Eat Before Bed?

Those three hours before sleep are a key element in helping your body wind down and prepare for the tasks it completes during sleep. During the REM sleep cycle, cerebral spinal fluid is pumped more quickly through the brain, acting like a "vacuum cleaner" to remove molecular detritus and toxic proteins that can build up in the brain in the course of daily living.

In this process of autophagy, activated primarily during sleep, brain cells eliminate damaged cell organelles and unused proteins, remove damaged mitochondria, and eradicate infectious particles. Studies have found that when the body is able to properly conduct autophagy it can inhibit the growth of cancer cells, prevent non-alcoholic fatty liver disease, and combat neurodegenerative diseases.

Allowing our bodies to complete the digestive process several hours before we sleep gives our brains the chance to focus on the autophagy process, as well as protects us from the melatonin-inhibiting effects of insulin secretion too close to bedtime. Better sleep makes for better autophagy, a "cleaner" brain and ultimately, a sharper mind.

Healing Foods for Your Brain

Eating less sugar is the first step to boosting your metabolism and recovering insulin sensitivity. The more sugar we consume, the more our addictive dopamine receptors call us, and the sweeter we need the next bite to be. Reducing, or ideally, removing all sources of added sugars allow our palate to reset and taste the natural sweetness in whole, natural foods.

As mentioned above, patients often tell me that within a few days of adopting a no-added-sugar diet, plentiful in cooked vegetables, proper protein intake, legumes, spices, fresh whole fruits, and healthy fats, etc., they no longer crave sugar at all. It takes a real shift in eating habits, but it's not the lifelong battle against temptation that you might imagine.

Sugar and Sweeteners

Controversy and confusion abound regarding the safety and glycemic effects of alternative sweeteners, which are commonly added to "health foods" instead of refined sugar. Before diving into the topic of "natural" sweeteners, I would like to put forth a general recommendation to avoid artificial sweeteners, as they are associated with increased rates of obesity and diabetes, even though they do not apparently provoke insulin response.

Cutting edge research from Ben-Gurion University of the Negev in Israel and Nanyang Technological University in Singapore may have revealed why. In their studies, *artificial sweeteners were shown to have a toxic effect on gut microbes*, effectively killing off beneficial strains and promoting obesity, elevated cholesterol and other blood lipids, and insulin resistance. Researchers tested the toxicity of aspartame, sucralose, saccharine, neotame, advantame, and acesulfame potassium-k, with similar results. Just one more reason to pass on the diet drinks and artificially sweetened *anything*!

In general, natural sweeteners, if they are organic and from whole food sources, are not unhealthy in and of themselves. Rather, it's how your body responds to them that counts, and that will vary by individual. Just as we saw above, identical foods with the same glycemic index can invoke very different blood sugar responses after consumption.

Long-term studies on the effect of regular consumption of natural sweeteners on insulin sensitivity and blood sugar control is lacking in most cases. However, they appear to be considerably safer than artificial sweeteners, including high fructose corn syrup. I recommend you avoid *all* added sweeteners, artificial or "natural," if you are trying to optimize your blood sugar and/ or cognition, with the possible exception of organic stevia (see below).

For an unbiased, evidence-based discussion and further guidance, I direct you to Dr. Thomas Guilliams' excellent book on sweeteners and other dietary nutrients, *Supplementing Dietary Nutrients, A Guide for Healthcare Professionals*. Today's online media is so filled with conflicting, "latest, greatest," and questionably sustainable "new wisdom," that it may be well worth your time and resources to invest in such a book, even if targeted to a professional audience, that is well-researched and presented from the practical perspective of a seasoned healthcare professional.

Now let's dive into some specific recommendations about several common natural sweeteners.

Agave. Pros: Usually organic and extracted from a whole plant, agave mainly contains naturally occurring fructose, which is relatively low in glycemic index (GI). However, actual GI depends on how much is consumed and to what food it is added. My recommendation: Agave may be occasionally consumed in small amounts if you have totally optimal fasting insulin, glucose, and HgA1C (part of your "Cognoscopy"; see Chapter Eight, Months One and Four). Avoid it if you are working on optimizing your glucose handling and following Ketoflex 12/3 to improve your cognition.

Fructose. "Fructose" is a non-specific term in today's market, as it may span the range of naturally occurring in fruit to artificially altered forms such as high fructose corn syrup. Here we are not considering the fructose you consume when eating whole fruit, which is fine.

Pros: "organic fructose" or fructose extracted from organic whole fruits and concentrated for addition to foods is theoretically healthful and OK, but only if used occasionally and in small amounts, according to your individual response, avoiding glycemic stress.

Cons: Paradoxically, although fructose, is "low glycemic index," it is associated with insulin resistance, obesity, metabolic syndrome, and diabetes. Moreover, most commercially sourced fructose is derived from cornstarch or sugar beets, which are usually genetically modified and subject to high levels of herbicide and pesticide residues, another potential source of endocrine disruption and damage to your sugar-handling system. I certainly recommend avoiding all fructose products that lack organic, non-GMO-verified status.

Polyols. Sugar alcohol molecules such as xylitol, sorbitol, mannitol, erythritol, and maltilol, generally have a low glycemic index. However, they are not as calorie-free as often advertised and can vary a lot amongst themselves. For example, while maltilol and xylitol have over 60 percent of sugar's calories per gram, erythritol has as little as 1/20th the calories. The rest fall somewhere in between.

The main caveat with polyols is that many people do not digest them well. Polyols are a FODMAP food (Fermentable Oligosaccharides, Disaccharides, Monosaccharides, and Polyols, which are short-chain carbohydrates and sugar alcohols that are poorly absorbed by the body), commonly creating gas and bloating. Be sure to avoid polyols if they are not non-GMO-verified as most are derived from corn. Today, nearly all corn is genetically modified and laden with toxins.

Stevia. This sweetener is extracted from the leaves of the *Stevia rebaudiana* plant and concentrated to form the non-nutritive white powdered sweetener many of us are familiar with.

Pros: Stevia can be as much as 300 times as sweet as sugar, gram per gram, yet studies indicate it elicits no insulin or elevated blood sugar response. There is no evidence to support the concept that the sweet taste in stevia may "trick the brain" into reacting as if you ate sugar. Long term studies are still limited, but short-term studies in both animals and humans indicate no adverse effect on the sugar-handling system, and even suggest glycemic improvement in some studies.

Cons: The main downside is that some people find stevia "bitter" tasting, rather than pleasantly sweet. Personally, I use stevia fairly often and, although at first it was not as appealing as the sugar taste I had grown up on, I now find it satisfying, and sugar-sweetened foods unattractively "too sweet."

In my personal and professional experience, the concept of "sweet begets craving for more sweet," while certainly true with respect to refined sugar, does not apply to stevia. If anything, stevia has a protective effect against the vicious cycle of sugar craving. If you have eschewed stevia and continued use of sweeteners that may stress your sugar-handling capacity, I recommend you give it another try. Brands like "Sweet Leaf" claim they are "without bitterness or aftertaste." My experience is that the taste of stevia has improved over the years, or at least, my taste buds have grown happier with it!

Food Choices To Favor

As you embark on optimizing your blood sugar, insulin sensitivity, and ability to "flex" into ketone burning during the 24-hour cycle, it is important to eat a relatively low carbohydrate diet with adequate (and not excessive) protein along with plenty of healthy fats. Avoid all refined, processed carbohydrates like muffins, bread, candy, cookies, cakes, pasta, white potatoes, processed foods, alcohol, any added sweetener other than stevia, and soft drinks.

Keep in mind that many so-called "protein bars" are high in carbohydrates and sugar and can promote blood sugar spikes as well as weight gain. One of my patients, Karin, age 67, eats five such bars a day, as her job in the operating room precludes regular meals with cooked vegetables, etc. She counts her calories and eats only organic bars, so she can't understand why she is gaining body fat and her fasting insulin is suboptimal. Inconveniently, as you recall, sugar consumption promotes fat deposition, as well as insulin resistance.

On the other hand, another patient of mine, Josephine, lost 35 pounds at age 64 "without trying," just by implementing regular, home-cooked meals with plenty of cooked vegetables, and substituting whole nuts and seeds for her prior protein bar snacks.

My suggestion: keep a stash of nuts, seeds, avocado and fresh fruits for your afternoon "snack attack," You may just effortlessly drop a few unwanted pounds as a side effect!

When choosing foods to prepare for meals or snacks, refer back to the Mediterranean Diet guidelines in Chapter Two and reach for:

- *Vegetables*. Choose mainly non-starchy vegetables, especially the detoxifying cruciferous ones such as broccoli, bok choy, cabbage, Brussels sprouts, and cauliflower. They are high in vitamin A, vitamin C, and K, minerals, dietary fiber, and folate. Fresh garlic is also a great choice for heart health, immunity and detox support.
- *Fruit*. Avoid juices, and even smoothies if they are not predominately protein- or vegetable-based. Rather, eat whole fruit, which is high in nutrients and fiber. Organic berries have been shown to protect the brain from changes associated with cognitive decline, and avocados provide a rich source of healthy fat, as well as providing a satisfying and filling snack or meal item.
- *Nuts and seeds*. High in nutrients, healthy fats, proteins, vitamins, and minerals, nuts should be part of everyone's regular diet. Choose raw and unsalted, and soak them overnight first, to eliminate "anti-nutrients" that interfere with digestion. Eat a variety of these powerful superfoods: flax, sesame, pumpkin, walnuts, almonds, Brazil

nuts, macadamia, and other seeds and nuts, all with their unique health benefits.

- *Legumes.* These are a great choice for vegans and vegetarians looking for protein and minerals. Legumes such as chickpeas, split peas, beans, lentils, mung dahl, urad dahl, and tamarind, are all useful but should be soaked overnight in water that is discarded before cooking, for maximum digestibility. Drizzling with fresh lemon or lime juice will help your body extract the minerals.

- *Animal protein.* Treat animal protein as a condiment and not the focus of a meal. Choose organic, grass-fed pastured, and high omega-3 sources. Eggs offer a rich source of choline, a micronutrient needed for the formation of acetylcholine, a primary neurotransmitter depleted in Alzheimer's Disease.

- *Oils.* Favor organic olive and avocado oils (the latter is heat resistant and especially good for cooking). Use MCT oil when needed to help your body make ketones. (See guidelines above.) Start with one-half teaspoon and increase to a maximum of one tablespoon three times a day. Other options for daily use are coconut oil or grass-fed ghee. Be cautious with the latter three, especially if you have the ApoE4 gene, as, like MCT oil, they are high in saturated fat and too much can accelerate atherosclerosis and amyloid plaque formation.

- *Herbs and spices.* There are a vast number of spices with a significantly wide range of benefits, including digestive support, helping regulate blood sugar, inhibiting amyloid formation, antioxidant, anti-inflammatory, anti-anginal and anti-carcinogenic effects, to name just a few.

See the end of this chapter for a chart of spices that help support carbohydrate metabolism, prevent neurodegenerative diseases, and reduce insulin resistance. See Chapter 7 for a Detox

Spice Mix, and Detox "Wise Water," a hot water infusion of fresh spices for detox and digestion-enhancing support.

You can add spices to tea, food, and salads; even soak them in hot water and drink as a customized infusion ("tea without the tea leaves") to readily absorb their unique benefits. I whole-heartedly encourage you to explore, experiment, and otherwise take advantage of these concentrated tasty packets of Nature's healing intelligence on a daily basis.

How Do You Know If You're Making Enough Ketones?

While working to stimulate ketosis and lower your blood sugar, it is important to monitor and test your levels. Testing your ketone levels will tell you if a "keto" food plan is working for you. Eating keto food doesn't automatically mean you are in ketosis. Ketosis is a measurable state of metabolism. This means you can test if your diet and daily fasting schedule is adequately ketogenic to allow your body to enter ketosis.

To keep it simple, I recommend that you first begin by measuring your fasting morning blood sugar. Once it's consistently below 90, you can also start testing your morning fasting ketone levels.

Note: You may have to keep adjusting your diet and trying different foods and timing of meals, as well as reducing your caloric intake to get your blood sugar down. One participant in the My Ageless Brain™ Online Course (*www.myagelessbrain.com*) wrote that she was struggling to get her morning blood sugar down. Finally, without changing what she ate, or how much, she simply ate her evening meal earlier, by 6:30 p.m., instead of 7:30 or 8 p.m. Bingo! Her morning fasting glucose was well below 90 for the first time.

Testing your glucose and ketone levels is really simple as long as you have a meter than measures both blood glucose and ketone levels. A suggested affordable brand is Precision Xtra meter, and there are many others available online. Follow the procedure described on the meter, pricking your finger and using the respective test strips to get your readings. Keep a record of your values.

When they have been in the optimal range, 0.5 to 4.5 for at least 2 weeks, you can stop measuring them every day, as long as you maintain the same diet and eating schedule. If you deviate due to travel, eating out, house guests, and so on, pull out your meter and test your values each morning. Remember that your brain and cognition will recover fastest if you stick with the program and only make exceptions when unavoidable.

Give yourself some time to get used to measuring—it will quickly become routine—and keep in mind that what works best to achieve optimal values varies from person to person. You may even respond very differently to the same food differently under different circumstances, such as excess stress, poor sleep, hormonal shifts, and many other factors. Identifying and addressing your triggers will help you adjust your diet and eating to keep your sugar in an optimal range in spite of the fluctuations of life. To "know thyself" in this regard and eat accordingly will provide a lasting boon to your brain health.

Cooking with Spices

Spices have long been used and studied in natural health. On the next page is a list of spices that are known to help blood sugar. Begin to use them regularly in your cooking, as teas (i.e., dissolved or infused in hot water) or as supplements. If you are taking medication to lower your blood sugar, monitor your levels carefully to ensure they don't go too low as a result of these herbs and spices. Consult your physician about adjusting your medication if your blood sugar drops significantly. If you make regular use of herbs and spices, you just might significantly improve insulin resistance and diabetes, the ideal end result!

The Healthy Brain Solution for Women Over Forty

Oregano	Oregano has been found to have one of the highest antioxidant levels of all the herbs and spices. It inhibits the formation of sugar-protein complexes called AGEs, implicated in Alzheimer's disease and measurable in the blood as hemoglobin A1C.
Cinnamon	Several studies demonstrate cinnamon's ability to lower fasting blood sugar and blood sugar after a meal.
Turmeric	Turmeric has been proven to turn off several blood sugar raising pathways in the body.
Garlic	In one study, subjects who ate raw garlic for 4 weeks saw a profound reduction in blood sugar, cholesterol, and triglycerides.
Gymnema sylvestre	This vine, native to India, has been shown to drastically reduce blood sugar levels—with some participants able to forego diabetes medication long-term as a result of regular use.
Fenugreek	Multiple studies show that fenugreek lowers blood sugar by slowing digestion and absorption of carbohydrates in the digestive system. Soak 2 teaspoons in water overnight, toss out the water in the morning and chew and swallow the softened seeds for greatest sugar-lowering effect.
Ginseng	Common in Chinese medicine for years, this potent herb has been shown to lower HgA1C levels, a measure of average blood sugar, over about 2 to 3 months.
Berberine	Sourced from the berberis shrubs, this potent hypoglycemic spice has effects comparable to Metformin, the prescription drug given to diabetics to lower blood sugar. Be sure to check with your doctor before taking if you are on medication or have a health condition, as berberine may strongly affect the metabolism of some medications.

Take This Simple Action #4 Now!

Go to *www.thehealthybrainsolution.com/sugar* and download your helpful guide on to how to "biohack" (measure directly) your blood sugar and keep your metabolism functioning at its "brain best." It's a lot simpler than you may think and will empower your optimal brain performance.

www.thehealthybrainsolution.com/sugar

5

Nourish Your Brain Back to Health

Let food be thy medicine and medicine be thy food.

—Hippocrates

Key #5: Correct Your Nutritional Deficiencies

We all know that wholesome food is a must for a healthy brain. As we've seen, fresh organic whole foods keep inflammation in check, support balanced sugar metabolism, reduce oxidation, and help our bodies detoxify. All good for brain, mind, and memory. But is it *enough*?

Lack of abundant nutrients and hormones can result in what has been called atrophic or "type 2 Alzheimer's." In type 2 (*vata type* according to Ayurveda), chronic lack of nutrition—vitamins, minerals, oils, proteins, as well as hormones—gradually damages the brain by depriving it of the nutrients and growth-promoting hormones it needs to thrive.

Type 2 patients often are thin and trim, do not have inflammation, and can even be athletic and seem the picture of health. They just can't remember what they ate, said, were told, or what happened yesterday, earlier in the day or even (at more advanced stages) five minutes ago. In this type of "amnestic" condition, the hippocampus usually shrinks first, disproportionately to the rest of the brain, leaving the mind's overall functioning fairly intact in the early stages, but short-term memory and learning seriously impaired.

Nutrients as "Trophic" or Growth Factors

As you may recall from Chapter One, the molecular precursor to amyloid, APP, is found in every nerve cell membrane. APP breakdown inherently triggers one of two critical pathways, determined by the state of the brain milieu. One pathway is destructive, leading nerve cells to shrivel and die while the other stimulates nerve growth, synaptic connections, and overall cell health and vitality.

Obviously, we want our brain cells to grow and thrive, so we need our APP molecules to be "cooperating" and not over-triggering amyloid production. Wouldn't it be great if our brains had a mechanism to block the amyloid-triggering pathway? It turns out they do! Growth-promoting molecules called "trophic" factors *bind* to the APP receptor and *prevent it from making amyloid and triggering cell death.* In this way, our brain cells *depend* on such molecules to stay healthy and alive, hence, APP is referred to as a "dependence" receptor, a type Bredesen himself and his colleagues discovered and coined.

In this and the next chapter, key "synapse-supporting" nutrients and hormones are described, each of which plays a role in *binding* to the APP molecule and *keeping* it *in* a mode of supporting healthy nerves, and *out* of the mode of creating amyloid. These nutrients and hormones, so-called brain growth or "trophic" factors, are needed in abundance to help keep amyloid production down and to prevent the nerve "shriveling" and death that happens all too quickly when there aren't enough of them around.

When Wholesome Food Is Not Enough

Unlike the experience of most doctors, the majority of my patients have been consuming wholesome, mainly organic, plant-based foods for decades. I've observed the many benefits of this way of eating. While not every patient is perfectly healthy, compared to the average population of patients and those I occasionally see in other settings, most of my patients have generally enjoyed good health, are free of serious chronic illnesses and, more often than not, have required no prescribed medication until their 60s, 70s, or beyond. With nearly 60 percent of the US population over age 20 taking at least one prescription medication regularly, and 15 percent taking five or more, the fact that most of my patient population have needed no regular medication, or only in their 60s or 70s, is a testament to the power of eating right, leading a balanced lifestyle and effectively reducing stress. (Many of them also practice meditation daily, most commonly Transcendental Meditation.)

On the other hand, in the face of dietary discretion, including but not limited to vegetarian and vegan diets, it is extremely important to ensure the adequate intake of all essential nutrients on an ongoing basis. In my vegetarian and vegan patients, nutritional deficiencies are all too common—especially when they don't take vitamin and mineral supplements—and can cause serious damage if not identified and corrected.

I've diagnosed and worked with thousands of patients to correct their nutritional deficiencies, such as B12 and the serious nerve damage that may have resulted, even in patients as young as 40 years old. In this chapter, I'm going to share with you the key nutrient deficiencies I see that contribute to brain and memory deterioration, and what you need to do to prevent them in yourself.

Are You Deficient?

The brain requires a tremendous amount of energy for its size. While it comprises only 2 percent of your body weight, it uses up to 20 percent of the body's energy, more than any other organ. I think we've all noticed how concentration, focus, and fluency can suffer if we are "running on empty," skipping or delaying meals, or eating junk food. Without fresh, wholesome foods on a regular schedule, the brain just doesn't get the nutrients it needs to perform at its best. Memory, focus, concentration, and creativity all begin to suffer, and mood swings may top it off.

I learned this the hard way a few years back. While I normally follow the Ayurvedic recommendation for regularity of mealtimes—and feel much better when I do—one day I was so engrossed in preparing for a radio show interview after lunch, that I didn't leave myself time to eat. While I got through the interview just fine, I distinctly noticed that my flow of speech was not as spontaneous as usual, required more effort and at times, the most articulate expression would elude me. After a nourishing snack brought me back to normal, I vowed to myself, "That's the *last* time I give a talk when I'm faint with hunger!" So far, I've kept my promise.

Prevention Power Tip—Test Thyself!

The number-one key preventive strategy I recommend you take is to undergo testing for a wide range of nutritional deficiencies that, if left untreated, can drain your brain power on a daily basis and leave you more vulnerable to Alzheimer's down the line. Knowing your results will help you get the most out of the seven keys to staying sharp you are learning in this book. You can readily remedy any deficiencies by following your personal physician's advice and go on to *optimize* beyond "normal" values using the guidelines in this chapter. (See Chapter Eight for a complete listing of tests I recommend.)

Correct Your Deficiencies

If you have a frankly abnormal value, it is imperative that you see your licensed medical practitioner and follow their advice on how to correct it. After treatment, you'll need to follow up with your doctor for a repeat blood test, to ensure your lab values have normalized and ideally, get them into an optimal range.

What Matters Most

Patients sometimes ask me, "Which nutrients matter the most—that I should be sure to check?" There is no simple answer to this. "Which nutrients matter most" is a very personal consideration. We just do not know what you might be low in. Once you get your results, the "ones that matter most" are the ones that are sub-optimal!

Do I Need to Supplement "Forever"?

Research corroborates that what you eat is crucial to the health of your brain. Yet I have found that, even in the most dedicated, health-conscious, and well-intended patients, those who are eating a variety of whole, organic foods with lots of fruits and vegetables, can still be low in nutrients. In a perfect world, no one would need supplements. However, because of the stresses of modern-day living, the poor quality of our food supply, our nutrient-depleted soils, and high levels of toxins in the environment, both wholesome foods *and* nutritional supplements are usually needed to optimize brain functioning.

I would also like to point out here *how important it is to continue to supplement on an ongoing basis after correcting a deficiency, though possibly at a lower dosage or frequency.* Unless you markedly change your diet on a consistent basis to provide the nutrients you were low in—or move to the beach and sunbathe daily without sunblock, in the case of Vitamin D—the great likelihood is that you will again get low in a nutrient when you stop supplementing it. This only sets you up for getting low again within the next few months to years—a risk you definitely want to avoid.

B12 Comes Back To Bite

For example, I have a subset of health-conscious, Baby Boomer patients who have been vegetarian since they were teenagers. They eat very similar diets and were diagnosed with low B12 in their late 30s or 40s. By that time, they had been vegetarian for about 20 years and had not taken B12 supplements. Once diagnosed with B12 deficiency, they dutifully *took* the supplements as recommended by their doctor and corrected their B12 blood levels, but eventually stopped taking them. (No one told them they would need to supplement for the rest of their lives.) Twenty years later, when I saw them in their 50s and 60s, many of them again had low B12 levels. But by now, decades of deficiency had taken a toll and neurological symptoms were common, and unfortunately, are reversible in only some of the cases.

Nutritional Risks: Take Measures to Avoid "Frailty"

I'm going to focus the following discussion of nutrients on two areas that I have seen are extremely important: first, vitamin B12 and second, adequate dietary protein. I've chosen to highlight these two because I see many patients who are deficient in one or both Such deficiencies are readily preventable, and it is imperative to prevent the damage and complications they can cause.

Let's consider protein intake first.

Inadequate dietary protein (and calories) is common in my patients who are underweight, lack physical strength and muscle mass, and may be careening downhill toward a medical condition termed "frailty," which is a strong risk factor for cognitive decline.

As a woman, you are one-third more likely to develop frailty than men of the same age. Adequate nutrition, including protein, vitamins, and minerals, along with weight- bearing exercise, is critical to prevent it. Our increased risk of frailty may explain some of the increased risks of Alzheimer's in women and is, fortunately, preventable.

One of my patients, who is now 70 and hasn't slowed down a bit, even in her retirement, explained to me that she long ago decided never to become a "little old lady," and has successfully pursued exercise, nutrition, and staying mentally and spiritually active as her path. I think we all share her desire to be healthy, vital, and strong "wise women" who stay "sharp as a tack." With a proper understanding of our body's needs and a commitment to meeting them, we can every day move closer to our strongest, most vital self and keep "frailty" and Alzheimer's at bay.

Now let's take a look at some of the winning, brain-healthy food and lifestyle strategies supported by research and clinical experience.

Eat Wholesome Proteins

Protein is an essential component of our daily diet. Our DNA expresses itself through the synthesis of protein. DNA gives its orders and guidance to the body through proteins, which are constantly being generated and broken down depending on the physiological needs of the body at any moment. Structurally, protein is an important building block for hair, nails, skin, bones, muscles, cartilage, and blood. We also need protein to make our enzymes, hormones, neurotransmitters, and many other cellular components.

We commonly hear that Americans eat too *much* protein. That may be true, or not, depending on which research you read. While experts debate the "right amount," it's important to realize that our personal need for protein can vary day by day depending on our exercise level, whether we are fighting an infection, recovering from surgery, traveling versus sitting at home, working hard on the computer or outside in the garden, or relaxing in our backyard. Life is dynamic, our bodies are ever adapting and so must our diet shift to match our needs.

Nonetheless, to get a rough idea, let's turn to the recommended daily allowance (RDA) for the "official answer," based on your body weight. To find out your RDA for protein, take your weight in pounds and multiply it by 0.36 (or your weight in kg × 0.8). The number you get is the number of grams of protein you should consume each day when you are not regularly exercising. This turns out to be about 50 grams for a 140-pound, sedentary woman. With exercise, protein needs increase, so if you are physically active, use 0.5 rather than 0.36 in the above calculation, which in this case would bring it up to 70 grams.

Experts point out that the RDA is generally set at the *minimum* needed to avoid getting a protein-deficiency disease and delivers about 10 percent of dietary calories as protein each day. The average American *does* consume more protein than that—about 16 percent dietary protein. The question then becomes "is that OK, or *too much?*" We are used to hearing that Americans consume as much as twice the protein that they should, yet recent research suggests 16 percent may be optimal, not excessive, and depends on your age, gender, and activity level.

To answer this question for *you*, I'm going to suggest that you reflect on your own diet, your level of health and vitality, and your life situation. If you feel basically strong, vital, and healthy, and eat mainly a plant-based diet with animal flesh foods and byproducts as a "condiment" rather than the *main meal* (think Chinese stir fry with a mound of vegetables speckled with smaller chunks of protein), you are probably eating the "right" amount for you.

Sources of Protein

Rather than get more hung up on how *much* protein you need, let's turn to the *sources* of protein you choose to fulfill your needs, whatever that amount may be.

If you are eating the "SAD" diet (Standard American Diet) with a generous portion of animal flesh as the main dish, such as red meat or pork, and your daily vegetable consists solely of the lettuce and tomato on your lunchtime sandwich, there's more to accomplish than just reducing protein.

It's time for an overhaul of how and what you're eating! Strive to align your diet with a Mediterranean-style diet rich in vegetables, olive oil, nuts, seeds, legumes, and mainly wild-caught, low-mercury fish as the animal protein source. The exciting thing is that adjusting your diet may not only help burn off brain fog but can boost you to a whole new level of health—free of aches, pains, morning lethargy, sinus problems, and a host of symptoms that commonly result from the pro-inflammatory SAD diet, not to mention lowering your cancer and Alzheimer's risk at the same time.

Foods High in Protein	
Food	Protein (grams)
3 ounces wild Alaskan salmon	21
3 ounces cooked organic turkey or chicken	19
6 ounces plain Greek yogurt	17
½ cup organic cottage cheese	14
½ cup cooked dried beans or other legumes	8
1 cup of organic milk	8
1 cup cooked pasta	8
¼ cup or 1 ounce of nuts (all types)	7
1 egg	6
Source: Adapted from the USDA National Nutrient Database, 2015	

The Power of Protein

Nan's Wisdom

In the kitchen one morning, during a week-long visit years ago, my mother-in-law Nan (bless her highly intelligent and caring heart) stopped in her tracks and said, as if a revelation just hit her, "I'm not sure you're getting enough protein." Of course, I, the doctor—and a nutritionally oriented one at that—was confident that she didn't know what she was talking about, plus was likely biased by her many decades of steak-and-potato meals. What could she possibly know about the adequacy of protein in my well-balanced, organic, whole foods, and mostly cooked at home, lacto-vegetarian diet? Harrumph! Of course, I politely assured her that I was getting plenty of protein and my diet was just fine, which I wholeheartedly believed.

Josie's Story—How Are Your Amino Acids?

Around that time, a nutritionist came to see me for some peri-menopausal issues. When I inquired about her diet, she commented that she wished she could be vegetarian and had tried it unsuccessfully in the past. She had low energy on it and was just not able to get as much done. A holistic nutritionist colleague of hers offered to test her *amino acid profile*, a simple blood or urine test that looks at the levels of all the amino acids (including the "essential" ones that your body can't make and needs to get from your diet).

Josie was shocked at the results. Her levels of essential amino acids—and many others—were appallingly low. No wonder she had been feeling low in energy! She didn't have the protein building blocks needed to make enzymes to run her metabolism, digest her food, detox chemicals, or keep her muscles, hair, skin, nails, and bones strong.

Without enough protein, her skin, hair, and body were aging and deteriorating faster? Indeed, it seemed that way. That did it! Josie immediately reintroduced free- range, grass-fed, organic meats into her diet, as well as occasional protein shakes when she exercised a lot. She said she felt so much better, she had never considered going vegetarian again, though she still wished—as an animal-lover at heart—that a vegetarian diet would work for her.

Over time, once recovered, she was able to reduce her intake of animal protein to mainly wild-caught fish, relying also on legumes, nuts, seeds, eggs, and some occasional goat dairy products to fulfill her protein needs. She also continued with unsweetened, organic protein shakes after workouts, and varies the protein type in hopes of not stressing her body with the same powder, day after day.

Note: I also recommend this strategy of rotating protein powders, just as you may rotate foods as part of a well-balanced whole foods diet with a wide variety of fruits and vegetables. Ayurveda describes that any food which is not in its natural synergy of components (such as in a protein isolate) is harder for the body to digest and use properly. Adding some cinnamon, ginger, cardamom, or turmeric to your shake is a good idea to support digestion, and it tastes great, too! Avoid cold water and don't mix in milk or yogurt to avoid hard-to-digest food combinations that leave you "heavy" in the stomach—not exactly the light and energetic feeling you want after exercise!

"Eat Meat or Die"

It was another year or so before Jim, a 58-year-old administrator, came to visit me. He had been vegetarian for over 40 years and was committed to continuing his vegetarian way of life. On his intake form, in answer to "what is the reason for your visit?" he wrote, "Am I getting enough protein?" Jim went on to say he'd been to his chiropractor recently, who looked at his thin frame and wan facial features and declared, "You must eat meat, or you will die!"

I took this to be a bit dramatic, but since Jim was obviously worried about it, and had come for my opinion, I felt compelled to answer it with the best objective data possible. Josie the nutritionist came to my mind, and I offered Jim, "We can test to see if you need more protein or not. A simple blood test will show us the level of amino acids in your blood and compare them to the norm. This will give us a good indication of whether you need to eat meat, or perhaps, add *other* sources of protein, even vegetarian ones."

Jim thought this was an excellent idea and we proceeded with the test. Indeed, the results showed a very low level of several essential amino acids, and many others. Compared to the general population, his levels were in the second percentile—meaning 98 percent of all people tested had higher levels of amino acids than Jim. Even if many of these other people ate "too much protein," Jim's markedly low levels, coupled with complaints of low stamina, exhaustion after exercising, and loss of much of his muscle mass since he had been a much more robust and athletic man in his 20s, indicated to me that more protein in his diet was in order.

I reassured Jim that I didn't believe his results meant he had to "eat meat or die," but I did recommend that he add another 25 to 30 grams per day of wholesome protein sources of his choosing. Jim was relieved, added concentrated plant-based protein sources, including organic cottage cheese, paneer (an Indian cheese he liked in curries), and a protein powder he liked and digested well. We also added more calories, and "healthy fats" to his diet, such as 2 or 3 tablespoons of organic olive oil at lunch daily, to help him gain some weight and "fill out" his frame. He started to go to the gym, upon my encouragement, and lifted weights twice a week, resulting in a gain of much-needed muscle mass, strength, and tone.

Jim successfully turned around his very slow, but steady decline towards "frailty" as he got older, a strong risk factor for shorter lifespan and a variety of chronic diseases, including the "atrophic" subtype of Alzheimer's disease.

By the way, Jim's test results prompted me to test amino acid profiles on nearly 100 of my vegetarian patients, including myself! I observed that patients who were following what was perhaps "too conscientious" a diet, with multiple self-imposed restrictions and without substantial concentrated protein sources such as eggs, dairy, or protein supplements, were usually low in amino acids and shared symptoms of suboptimal vitality similar to Jim's. Increasing their protein intake, as I had advised Jim, turned their symptoms around fairly quickly.

Some patients elected to add back the fish and poultry they had eaten earlier in their lives. Ironically, several patients remarked to me that they had *better* spiritual experiences and meditation since returning to chicken or fish, even though they had adopted vegetarianism to support their yoga practice and their spiritual development. That was no surprise to me. Since protein is the building block of major neurotransmitters in the brain, it's no wonder that providing better "fuel" to brain cells could result in better meditation. After all, every experience we have—whether sacred or mundane—is an expression of brain chemistry, and food runs our biochemical engine.

Nan's Wisdom—Follow-up

In case you're wondering, my mother-in-law was right. My amino acids, and many minerals and vitamins, were low. That was 20 years ago. I have since made a conscious effort every day to include adequate protein (vegetarian with rare exceptions), and take my organic multi-vitamin, minerals, and extra B vitamins. As an aside, woman-to-woman, I have noticed that how fresh or youthful I look has a lot to do with how much nutrition I'm getting—in addition to an early bedtime, good sleep, a morning walk outdoors—my anti-aging secrets!

B12

B12 is an essential B vitamin that nerve cells need to produce *myelin*, a fatty substance that coats a neuron's "arms and legs" (dendrites and axons) like insulation, protecting the nerve and speeding transmission of an electrical signal from one end of the neuron to the other. While not every neuron is myelin-coated, most of the axons in the central nervous system are, and speed of transmission (like your speed of thinking, among other functions) relies on it. Demyelination due to B12 deficiency can lead to memory loss over time, as well as anxiety, depression, numbness, tingling, balance problems, confusion, and dementia—damage that is not always reversible.

B12 deficiency is a very serious condition with potentially devastating long-term consequences. And yet, most doctors do not think to check for it, even in their high-risk patients, until *after* memory or nerve problems have already been diagnosed. Then it's too late for prevention. For a non-neurologist, I've seen and treated an inordinate amount of B12 deficiency cases, having cared for thousands of vegetarian and vegan patients over several decades.

I want to highlight the importance of B12 in hopes of preventing you, and many like you, from falling into the dismal abyss that B12 deficiency can carve in your brain.

Josephine's Story—Why Can't I Think?

Josephine is a married interior designer and co-owner and rental property manager who came to see for help recovering her brain following severe B12 deficiency diagnosed over 10 years before. I'll let Josephine tell her story:

As an interior designer, passionately committed to my successful career, I first noticed I was in trouble when I sat in front of a client's large window for 2 hours and could not estimate the drapery yardage of a design that I was envisioning for that window. When I tried to calculate an estimate for another large design job, it took me hours to do the calculations. I spent half the night at it. I felt like something had happened to my brain. It felt like a heavy anvil was on my brain and my brain was incapable of transmitting the information that I needed.

The heavy "iron anvil" experience would appear whenever I tried to estimate, as if that brain passage had shut down. I began to avoid estimates, purchase orders, and anything to do with calculations. I had 13 rentals in three different cities, a full-time interior design business with six to twelve projects going at once, including a 24-foot exhibition at a large, world-class museum, taught meditation on the side, and cooked three wholesome meals a day for my busy, working husband.

The sudden additional pressure of an unexpected project dropping on me caused all parts of my life to crumple. I had serious burnout, mental overload, and, eventually, a mental "breakdown."

I suffered for two years without knowing why. I could not spell or write correctly, add or write numbers correctly, speak without slurring and had very slow word finding. I could not remember where I put my coat or my fabrics at my clients' home (or if I had put shampoo in my hair), could not remember where I was driving. I could not organize my files, could not learn how to use a computer, could not write a purchase order, and could not follow sequential instructions.

I thought I had "premature dementia" and would lose everything—my husband, home, career, everything I had worked for and that was precious to me. I could imagine another woman in my home with my husband, wearing my lovely jewelry and silk clothing, while I was in a "home" for persons with dementia.

I remember sitting in our car in our parking lot and realizing that I had to give up my interior design career after 30 years. Who was I if I was not an interior designer? I was totally identified with my designer career ... and now it was over.

I finally saw my primary doctor, who ordered a panel of tests, which did not include B12. (She herself, I later learned, was burned out and had her own B12 deficiency!)

As she had no answers for me, I asked to see a neurologist. She diagnosed me with "premature dementia," and asked to see my blood work. I thought that I had all the blood tests covered. The neurologist wisely said she should look at my blood tests for herself. She discovered that the B12 test was not included. It was an "aha" moment of possible hope and solution for me. The neurologist immediately ordered a B12 blood test.

My B12 level was under 200, which was very low. The neurologist prescribed B12 shots once a week for a month and thereafter, daily tablets to dissolve under the tongue. After taking the B12 shots, I immediately experienced positive change as in "Lazarus rising from the dead." It was if the lights went on in a previously blurry darkness of hopeless frustration.

Now, twenty years later, I've recovered much of my cognitive capacity, but some things have never come back. I have limitations I didn't before. Several months later, after the B12 injection treatments, I again tried to do a large design project. I became exhausted with the administration details, and a familiar confusion took over. I could feel myself going downhill and knew I could no longer take on big design projects.

Even now, I can get overwhelmed with paperwork and so my now-retired husband looks after the rentals.

It is a challenge to change brain channels and focus. It is as if I need a runway absolutely clear of pressure or interference in order to intensely focus. I often need to wear Bose headphones to block out interfering sounds, in order to help me focus. If I am speaking and someone interrupts me, I easily get derailed, which is frustrating.

I need to catch my creative ideas and thoughts like "netting a fish" or I may not ever have access to them again. I need to keep many notes on my ideas and keep "to do" lists as cues for my daily direction. There are still simple computer maneuvers that I cannot seem to manage to perform, like creating an attachment document. I also found I was unable to follow directions in a sequence while learning the hula dance. After 3 years, I gave it up for more spontaneous dance movements.

I still take B12 daily and maintain a high normal blood level. If I miss even a day, I feel it. In addition to B12 tablets, I have found the rejuvenation of Transcendental Meditation for 20 minutes twice a day to be extremely valuable. TM helps my brain to reset, rest and recharge. A regular routine of twice daily meditating, first thing in the morning and again in mid to late afternoon, has proven to be a healthy practice that my brain needs for maximum support. If I delay meditating until too late at night, I notice that I am not functioning as well.

Also, going to bed late diminishes my brain ability. If I get to bed before 10 p.m., I notice a difference in quality, freshness, and ease of brain functioning and daily organizing the next day. When I do not follow this routine, there is word searching and prolonged effort on any task. I also notice that too much time on the computer and not enough time walking or outdoors in nature adversely affects my brain functioning.

Listening to certain Vedic chants is helpful to my brain. I noticed that I could estimate much better and handle numbers after 6 weeks of listening to Vedic chanting for 10 minutes twice a day.

I also need to stay away from "the whites" — white sugar, white flour. If I have anything sweet, I notice that my brain becomes ungrounded. I am focusing on a "ketosis diet" — a good, healthy, oil-based diet to feed my brain. My breakfast mainstay is steamed vegetables sprinkled with "Dr. Nancy's Custom Smart Spice," ground seeds and nuts, a spritz of fresh lime juice, fresh herbs, and avocado if available, light on the Himalayan salt and pepper ... and a drizzle of olive oil.

The B12 deficiency is now behind me. Even with some lingering limitations, I am gratefully enjoying vibrant good health and a wonderful, purposeful, and conscious life.

Test and Optimize Your Nutrients

The B Vitamins:

A 2013 study showed that B vitamin supplementation slows brain shrinkage, specifically in brain regions known to be most severely affected by Alzheimer's disease. The shrinkage was decreased by as much as seven-fold! Vitamins B6, B9 (folate), and B12 are three B vitamins that essential for brain health. Sufficient levels of those three vitamins are needed to keep homocysteine levels in check. Homocysteine is a by-product of metabolism and a well-known cardiovascular risk factor that is damaging not only to the arteries, but also the bones and the brain.

Now let's take a look at each individually:

Vitamin B12

While we've already talked a lot about B12, there are a few more points worth knowing. Nearly two-fifths of the U.S. population may be flirting with marginal vitamin B12 status if the population of Framingham, Massachusetts, is any indication. A careful look at 3,000 men and women in the ongoing Framingham Offspring Study found 39 percent with plasma B12 levels in the "low normal" range—below 258 picomoles per liter. The results were surprising. The youngest group—the 26- to 49-year-olds— had about the same B12 status as the oldest group—65 and up. "We saw a high prevalence of low B12 even among the youngest group," Tucker said.

Many are deficient in B12, especially if they are vegetarian or over 60. Vitamin B12 in its active form (methyl cobalamin) is crucial in keeping the brain and nervous system functioning optimally. It is needed for maximizing capacities in memory, focus, clarity, and concentration, and in preventing fatigue. Deficiency in vitamin B12 can lead to anemia and dementia.

Vitamin B12 must be ingested, as our body does not make it. It is present primarily in animal products, such as meat, poultry, fish, eggs, and dairy products. While chlorella may carry bioavailable forms of B12 as well, the amount is very small and varies widely from sample to sample. It is certainly not enough to correct a deficiency, and it may or may not be sufficient to prevent developing one when taken on a daily basis.

An important note: don't run out and start taking B12 before you check your blood level. Even one tablet of B12 may be enough to raise your blood level to the normal range, so it may mask deficiency that still exists in your body and you will never know if you were or are truly deficient. Why is that important? First of all, because deficiency can take as long as one year of daily supplementation to restore stores of B12 in your liver and other organs. And you are likely to get low again quickly if you stop this new supplement habit and were low to begin with.

Even more importantly, I've noticed it seems to be human nature to lose interest in taking a supplement if you don't know if you really need it or not. That can be dangerous if you are deficient in a vitamin as critical as B12.

My advice is to *resist* your enthusiastic impulse to start popping B12 tablets right now—go get your B12 blood test first. If you're low, you will be more likely to stay the course to fully correct your deficiency, and remember, you'll need to take it for life to prevent getting low again.

Vitamin B9 (Folate)

Vitamin B9 (folate) is required for a multitude of bodily functions including DNA synthesis and repair, cell division, and cell growth. Folate deficiency increases dementia risk, and no wonder. MRI findings show that the brain *atrophies* without it. Folate deficiency is also associated with depression. It affects mood and cognitive function, especially in older people, although it is important for the functioning of the nervous system at all ages. Taking methylfolate along with vitamin B12 in its methylcobalamin form, can increase the effectiveness of antidepressants, and with B6 (ideally in pyridoxyl-5-phosphate form) and other methyl donors like betaine or TMG (needed by some, depending on their genetics), can lower harmful homocysteine as well.

High-folate foods include beans, lentils, asparagus, spinach, broccoli, avocado, mango, lettuce, sweet corn, oranges, and whole wheat bread. Daily supplementation with 0.5 to 1.0 mg of methylfolate is usually adequate to correct a deficiency, but follow-up testing is needed to be sure.

Vitamin B6

Vitamin B6 is needed for proper brain development in children and brain function for people of all ages. It helps the body make the hormones serotonin, which regulates mood, and norepinephrine, which helps your body cope with stress. Your blood level for B6 should be between 60 to 100 nanomoles per liter—the upper limit because high levels can be toxic to your nerves, just as low levels can be damaging. Vitamin B6 is particularly synergistic with magnesium. The absorption of both elements is increased in the presence of the other. The best sources of vitamin B6 include meat, fish, poultry, organ meats, enriched cereals and non-GMO soy products, nuts, lentils, and some vegetables and fruit.

According to the Bredesen ReCODE program, the goal from your blood test results should be: B12 = 500-1500 pg/ml; folate = 10-25 ng/ml; B6 = 60-100 mcg/L.

Vitamin B1

Thiamine (vitamin B1) was the first B vitamin discovered by scientists. Like the other B vitamins, it is water-soluble. Thiamine

134

enables the body to use carbohydrates as energy. It is essential for glucose metabolism and normal system function. Some people use thiamine for maintaining a positive mental attitude; enhancing learning abilities; increasing energy; fighting stress; and preventing memory loss, including Alzheimer's disease. Thiamine helps decrease the risk and symptoms of a specific brain disorder called Wernicke-Korsakoff syndrome (WKS). This brain disorder is related to low levels of thiamine (thiamine deficiency) and is often seen in alcoholics.

B1 deficiency can be characterized by fatigue, muscle cramps, various pains, and reduced tolerance to pain, all factors that could be associated with dysmenorrhea (painful menstruation) and PMS.

Vitamin B2

Riboflavin (vitamin B2), is the only vitamin that gives you a visual cue about its passage through your body. When there is a lot of vitamin B2 in the diet (or in a supplement), your urine turns bright yellow to show you it is there. Riboflavin (vitamin B2) supports cellular energy production. It is involved in many processes in the body and is necessary for normal cell growth and function. Deficiency of riboflavin is rare in developed countries because it is a vitamin found in many common foods.

People eating a standard Western diet receive about one-quarter to one-third of their dietary vitamin B2 from milk and other dairy products. It can be found in leafy green vegetables, cauliflower, and Brussels sprouts, peppers, root vegetables, squash, eggs, nuts, and meat. Riboflavin is frequently used in combination with other B vitamins in vitamin B complex products.

Vitamin D: The Sunshine Vitamin

Your body must have vitamin D to absorb calcium. It helps build bones and keep bones strong and healthy. Vitamin D deficiency is very common these days because most people work and play indoors. Suboptimal vitamin D is associated with cognitive decline, depression, and dementia. How do you increase your level of vitamin D? The two main ways to get vitamin D are by exposing your bare skin to sunlight for twenty minutes per day, year-round, or by taking vitamin D supplements. Of course, most of us women today avoid exposing our skin to direct sunlight, to prevent skin cancers and premature aging. One alternative that works well for many women is walking outdoors, with face and hands exposed, before 9 or 10 a.m., when the sun is less direct, and the full benefits of outdoor morning sunlight can be gained.

Many patients ask me if they can get more vitamin D from food. Unfortunately, vitamin D3, the more effective form, is mostly absent from our food supply. (It's the D2 form that's typically added to milk and other foods.)

However, there are a few food sources that contain some vitamin D3 such as the fatty fish tuna, mackerel, and salmon, and egg yolks (easy to remember, they look like the sun!).

To maintain optimal blood levels, a daily intake of 1,000 to 4,000 IU or 25 to 100 micrograms is usually needed, a level considerably higher than the widely stated RDA of 400 IU per day. It may seem like a lot, but I have a number of patients who need to take 5,000 IU/day just to maintain an optimal blood level of vitamin D.

It is important to test your level of vitamin D3 as a baseline, and again a couple of months later, if you begin to supplement or increase your supplementation. Also, check it yearly to ensure your supplementation is keeping up with your body's need, as that can change over time. You should aim for a vitamin D level between 50 and 80 ng/ml and ensure that your daily vitamin D intake plus sunlight exposure maintains it in the optimal range over time.

Importance of Minerals for Your Brain

Balance in all phases of life is important to maintain health and this applies to mineral levels. What is a mineral ratio? A pure number consisting of one mineral level divided by a second mineral level. Mineral ratios are often more important than levels in determining nutritional deficiencies and excesses. Ratios represent homeostatic balances. They can frequently predict future or hidden metabolic dysfunctions.

The Copper:Zinc Ratio

Zinc deficiency is prevalent throughout the world and especially in older people. Too much copper and too little zinc are associated with depression and dementia. In fact, aging is associated with lower zinc levels. People with the toxic subtype 3 of Alzheimer's often have very low zinc levels. A study by Brewer et al. on the effects of copper and zinc on cognitive function found that most people are deficient in zinc and have excess copper. Zinc supplementation has been shown to enhance cognition.

The goal you should aim at in measuring your levels of copper and zinc in a blood test should be around 100 mcg/dL, a copper:zinc ratio of 1:1. Ratios of 1.4:1 or higher have been associated with dementia.

Sources of Zinc

Beans and legumes. This includes non-genetically modified foods (non-GMO) such as tofu, tempeh, black and green soybeans, kidney beans, black beans, garbanzo beans, lentils, and peanuts.

Nuts and seeds
Dairy products
Oats, wheat germ, nutritional yeast, whole grains, fortified cereals
Red meat and poultry, seafood

Sources of Copper

In my clinical experience, I rarely see copper deficiency. Usually, copper is around the "normal" level or higher, and zinc is the one disproportionately low. Without finding a deficiency in copper by a lab test, I do not recommend adding foods with copper to your diet, as you probably have enough already, and adding more will just tip the scales more out of balance in relation to zinc.

That said, here are some rich sources of copper, if you are in need it: oysters and other shellfish, whole grains, beans, nuts, potatoes, and organ meats (like kidney and liver). Less plentiful in copper, but still good sources are dark leafy greens, dried fruits such as prunes, cocoa, black pepper, and yeast.

Magnesium

Magnesium is critical for brain function. It is responsible for 300 enzyme reactions in your body used for regulating muscle and nerve function, blood sugar levels and blood pressure, and making protein, bone, and DNA. Most people are deficient in magnesium and it causes a long list of problems, from anxiety, insomnia, ADHD, and dementia. When a person has Alzheimer's, there is a great probability that the brain structures related to memory are low in magnesium.

What is the best kind of magnesium?

A randomized, controlled, double-blind study published in the *Journal of Alzheimer's Disease* concluded that nutritional supplementation with magnesium threonate (as Magtein® from AIDP), was effective at reversing cognitive impairment, and returned cognitive function almost back to normal ability relative to age. Considered one of the leading experts in magnesium and cognitive health, Liu was the principal investigator on the study. Magtein is a compound designed to help magnesium cross the blood-brain barrier, support an increase in brain synapse density and help restore cognitive abilities. This form of magnesium is especially good for neurological issues, brain injuries, depression, anxiety, and PTSD.

To achieve a level of magnesium optimal for brain function, you may need to add a magnesium supplement to your diet. Measuring the levels of magnesium in your red blood cells produces a more accurate reading than measuring it in serum. The test is called RBC (red blood cell) magnesium. The optimal goal for RBC magnesium is between 5.2 to 6.5 mg/dL.

Sources of magnesium

- Whole wheat. Most whole grains are a good source of magnesium, but whole wheat flour contains the most. Of course, it also contains gluten, so avoid this if you may be intolerant.
- Spinach and other dark, leafy greens are rich in magnesium. Add a squeeze of fresh lemon or lime juice to help your body assimilate the minerals.
- Quinoa
- Almonds, cashews, peanuts
- Black beans and edamame

Selenium

Selenium is a key mineral because it functions in a number of critical systems in the body that control proper mood and brain function. Selenium is required for thyroid function and is important in heavy metal detoxification. It also enhances immune system function. Deficiency in selenium has been shown to be associated with cognitive decline.

Seven of the best vegetarian sources of selenium

- Brazil nuts. They are one of the best sources of selenium!

- Shiitake/white button mushrooms
- Lima/pinto beans
- Chia seeds
- Brown rice
- Seeds (sunflower, sesame, and flax)
- Broccoli, cabbage, spinach.
- The goal for your blood test results should be: serum selenium = 110-150 ng/ml.

Herbal Superstars for Your Brain

Gotu kola (*Centella asiatica*). Gotu kola is a traditional Ayurvedic herb which research suggests is effective for improving memory, learning, and focus. In addition, gotu kola has exhibited anti-amyloid effects in animal studies. Other studies show calming and antidepressant activity, comparable to imipramine (a common antidepressant before Prozac came on the scene) and reduction of the "acoustic startle" response—i.e., startling in response to a sudden loud noise—providing evidence that it reduces anxiety. It is used traditionally for memory enhancement, as a sedative nervine, as a sleep aid and as an antispasmodic. It is considered to be a "balancing tonic" that both increases energy and relaxes the body.

Personally, I frequently enjoy tea made of gotu kola and tulsi (see below), which I find—unlike the buzz of caffeine—helps me focus while it enhances alertness and inner calm, all at the same time.

Bacopa (*Bacopa monnieri*). Also referred to as Brahmi or water hyssop, is a perennial plant used in Ayurveda and herbal medicines. *Note:* Avoid confusing Brahmi (*bacopa monnieri*) with gotu kola and other herbs that are also sometimes informally referred to as "brahmi." Research on Brahmi for the brain supports Brahmi's role as an antioxidant, anti-inflammatory, and in promoting acetylcholine levels, supporting thinking, learning, and memory. Brahmi also protects nerve cells from the damaging effects of beta-amyloid. Brahmi has been used for Alzheimer's disease, improving memory, anxiety, attention deficit-hyperactivity disorder (ADHD), allergic conditions, irritable bowel syndrome, and as a general tonic to fight stress.

Ashwagandha (*Withania somnifera*). Ashwagandha is a plant that is beneficial for its root and berry. It is used as an "adaptogen" to help the body cope with daily stress, supports thyroid function (whereas it is contraindicated in overactive thyroid conditions), and is regarded as a general tonic. Research indicates that ashwagandha calms anxiety, improves learning and memory, supports acetylcholine levels in the brain, promotes the formation of new neuronal connections, helps the regeneration of neurons, interferes with amyloid formation, and helps protect neurons from its toxic effect. Overall, ashwagandha is a "superstar herb" for the brain.

Holy basil or "tulsi" (*Ocimum sanctum*). The leaves, stems, and seeds of this plant that originated from India are used in Ayurvedic medicine as an "adaptogen" to counter life's stresses and relieve anxiety. It helps to lower excess cortisol, is anti-inflammatory, and supports a balanced immune response.

Note: It is important to evaluate the company and products you are going to buy. You should select products that have been tested for heavy metal contamination and bacteria (if they are from India or China in particular) and that are, ideally, organic and certainly non-GMO. You can research this yourself or enlist the help of an informed healthcare practitioner or nutritionist to select the best products for you.

A Few Key Brain Supplements

There is a plethora of supplements touting benefits for the brain, and indeed, many that have been shown, at least in the laboratory, to be of potential benefit to the brain and cognition.

In my practice, it is not uncommon for patients to come to me with cognitive complaints who are already taking a dozen or more supplements promoted as benefiting memory and cognition. However, most of those patients report that they have not noticed that any supplement in particular, or even the sum total of all the supplements, have made any appreciable impact on their memory or cognition.

In these memory loss patients, I have observed that supplements for the brain (i.e., above and beyond those specific nutrients given to correct an identified deficiency) give noticeable benefit only when the underlying causes of Alzheimer's—inflammation, glycotoxicity, nutrient deficiencies, hormone deficiencies, and toxic exposures—are also being corrected. In this context, adding a specific supplement may suddenly be correlated with a boost of mood, energy, focus, and even memory.

Leading practitioners using Bredesen's protocol have shared with me that they, too, aim to identify and correct all underlying causes first. Then, after those are established, they add in targeted supplements chosen for the individual depending on their specific needs.

Below, I share two common supplements that reduce inflammation and may help inhibit amyloid plaque formation, curcumin and resveratrol. A third, citicoline, performs a function similar to common anti-Alzheimer's drugs and has induced a noticeable memory boost in a few of my patients.

Curcumin is a powerful anti-inflammatory, antioxidant, and anti-amyloid molecule derived from turmeric root, a relative of ginger. Turmeric has been used for thousands of years as a medicinal preparation. For years, researchers have hypothesized that the very low rates of Alzheimer's in Indian villagers eating a traditional diet may be at least in part due to the generous 2 teaspoons or more of turmeric they use daily in their cooking. The compound that gives the popular Indian spice curry its mustard yellow color may indeed ward off Alzheimer's disease. Numerous studies have shown that the curry pigment curcumin powerfully slows the formation of, and even destroys, accumulated beta-amyloid plaque deposits in mouse brains.

While 1 gram twice a day is recommended, as curcumin or turmeric powder, on an empty stomach or with healthy oils, Ayurvedic tradition would have you add turmeric powder to all your cooking. I do this myself, as it has so many salutary properties. Not sure you like the flavor? Just use a little in many of your dishes, and you will not find it changes the flavor appreciably, yet it significantly enhances the brain protective power of your meal.

Resveratrol is part of a group of compounds called polyphenols. They're thought to act like antioxidants, protecting the body against damage that can put you at higher risk for cancer, heart disease, diabetes, and Alzheimer's. It has gained a lot of attention for its reported anti-aging and disease-fighting powers. It may protect nerve cells from damage and fight the beta-amyloid plaque buildup that can lead to the disease. More research is needed, but it shows potential for preventing and recovering from cognitive decline.

Citicoline (also known as CDP-choline) is a naturally occurring compound and a building block of cell membranes. The "choline" part is a nutrient similar to B vitamins and made by the liver. Citicoline is a common ingredient in supplements marketed for brain support. In Alzheimer's disease, choline levels decrease, reducing the brain cell's ability to produce acetylcholine, a neurotransmitter important for memory. Brain cells may instead break down cell membranes to produce acetylcholine; taking citicoline is thought to prevent this breakdown. It has no known side effects, unlike most prescription drugs for the same purpose.

Most prescription medications for Alzheimer's disease block the breakdown of acetylcholine, allowing more of it to build up in the gaps between cells, and improving cell-to-cell messaging. Termed acetylcholinesterase-blockers, they are used to treat mild to moderate dementia and often result in transient improvement in cognition lasting several months before cognitive abilities begin to drop off again. These drugs are, unfortunately, not a cure. They temporarily reduce symptoms but do not remove the underlying causes of Alzheimer's. While many patients tolerate them well, common side-effects include appetite loss, weight loss, insomnia, muscle cramps, tiredness, drowsiness, dizziness, weakness, shakiness, itchy skin, nausea, vomiting, or diarrhea.

A Promising Treatment Trifecta

A lesser known, but extremely beneficial triad of supplements has been shown to enhance memory as well as promote the production of phosphatidylcholine, a critical component of synapses and membranes in the brain. It turns out that our brain enzymes do a much better job of making cellular components when there are plenty of the necessary ingredients around. (Makes perfect sense—how do you make a walnut loaf when you're fresh out of walnuts?)

Researchers have found a triplet of ingredients that seems to hit the "sweet spot" for synaptic synthesis—the memory-critical connecting points between neurons. The omega-3 fatty acid DHA, choline, and uridine-5'-monophosphate (a constituent of RNA and involved in enzyme synthesis).

Taking the three together boosts activity of the enzymes that make synaptic membranes and appears to support cognition and memory in that way. If you are experiencing memory lapses, you may want to be sure you are including all three of these in your supplement regimen and see if taking them all regularly makes a difference for you. (As always, check with your doctor if you are taking medication or have a medical condition.)

Seeking "Supercognition"? A Sampling of Supplements to Enhance Memory and Performance

For those with basically good cognitive function who are looking for better name-recall and word-finding—two memory functions that tend to drop off with age—I'll mention two products that patients have shared have made a difference for them. It is a very short list, unfortunately, in spite of many products they (and I) have collectively tried for enhancing cognitive performance. These do not necessarily represent the only ones patients have told me have helped them, but they are the ones I have heard repeatedly from numerous patients over time. While not proven effective in controlled trials, the individual ingredients have all been shown to benefit the brain, mind, or memory.

One is the herbal product, "Youthful Mind™" by VPK, at *www.mapi.com*. It features the herbal "superstar," amyloid-busting gotu kola, presented above, along with synergistic herbs for the brain and for liver detox. Patients over the years have repeatedly reported to me that Youthful Mind™ helps their memory and focus.

The second product is also a proprietary combination, called "Protandim," a multi-level marketed product that initially I was very skeptical of, even though a trusted colleague claimed it made a big difference in her memory. Since then, however, I have seen it make a noticeable impact in an unprecedented number of people, even within a few days, as in, "Where did all those forgotten names suddenly come from?!" It contains turmeric, green tea extract, ashwagandha, and milk thistle—a combination product that, like Youthful Mind™, aims at detox and liver support as well as neuronal enhancement. Since its action can be so quick, if it doesn't help within 1 to 2 months, it may not be for you.

Other positive reports have come from patients of mine taking Bacopa consistently for several months, and from grapeseed extract.

Everyone is different, and you may find an entirely different supplement makes a positive difference for you. I tend to prefer herbal combinations over the long run, as they are inherently closer to food than are isolated ingredients and theoretically less likely to give side-effects. If you *don't* notice a benefit after taking an over-the-counter brain supplement (not to correct a specific deficiency), I generally recommend that you discontinue it, and keep up only those that you truly notice a benefit from. If you are following this protocol, you may already be taking a sizeable number of supplements to correct deficiencies found on your blood testing. Taking extra supplements can be counter-productive, in my opinion, adding extra load on your gut, liver, and kidneys to process and eliminate them.

In Summary

Atrophic Alzheimer's disease is commonly the end result of decades of insidious nutritional deficiency and hormonal insufficiency. As a woman over the age of 40, I encourage you to do the following:

First: Test your blood levels of the nutrients listed in this chapter.

Second: Optimize your blood levels with diet and supplements if a deficiency is detected.

Nourishment for The Feminine Soul

And finally: I have one more recommendation, which is subtler, yet perhaps as powerful as nutrient levels, supplements, and food itself, and has to do with a general regard and feeling that you may have already, or can culture, towards your body.

We women all too often have felt unkindly toward our bodies, transferring to *them* the messages we all too often glean, even subconsciously, from the media—we're not thin enough, we are not sexy enough, or pretty enough, or … we likely each have our own complaints about our bodies. Now, it's time to change all that.

I encourage you to begin to regard your body with appreciation, with love, with caring and compassion. Think of all the wonderful things it does, endlessly, every day, for *you.* Due to constant whirring of your nerve cells, you can think, and plan, share, communicate and love. Due to the perpetual beating of your heart, your cells are nourished and provided with the energy you need to get through the day alive, and hopefully, well. Your emotional heart, in communication with your brain, allows you refined feelings of love, compassion, joy, and happiness.

So, I entreat you, as a sister, a woman, a doctor, and your friend, please consider treating your body as the temple that it is, the sacred home of your soul on earth. Consider for a moment, your food as a gift to you from Mother Earth, who lovingly wants, like every mother, to nourish you and keep you healthy. Write in your journal, share with your female friends, how you are taking steps to nourish and heal your body not only physically, but with a deeply healing sense of appreciation, wonder, and gratitude.

I have no data on this, but I wanted to share from my heart that you are *special*, you are *important*, and it is wise to appreciate and care for yourself on all levels. You will give back more to the world and those you love, when you first care, now, for yourself.

While this mindset may seem unscientific, research does validate that gratitude and thankfulness are associated with better health. I personally believe we eat all too unconsciously and without due regard to the gift of wholesome, life-bestowing nutrition. We rush our meals, eat distractedly and all too often shove nearly anything in our mouths to keep going. Consuming even nutritious food in this setting may not benefit us as it should, as our "fight or flight" response compromises our digestion and assimilation. Rather, after eating, strive to "rest and digest," enlisting the full support of your parasympathetic nervous system, the obligate "conductor" of your miraculous digestive symphony.

As we close this chapter on nutrients for your brain, I encourage you to eat and prepare your food with reverence to yourself and the rich, organic earth that grew it, rich in essential nutrients for your brain and body. Avoid rushing your meals, eating on the run, skipping meals, and generally disregarding your body's need for a calm, settled environment for proper assimilation.

Rather, it's now time to follow the "zen" of eating—a path of gratitude, self-awareness, and even spiritual fulfillment for you, your body, and your precious brain. Eat mindfully and thankfully, taking in all the nutrients your brain and body need, and Mother Nature with her infinite healing power, will take care of the rest.

Take This Simple Action #5

Check out VPK Products for superstar
Ayurvedic herbs for brain health, including bacopa.

Their Youthful Mind™ formula contains gotu kola
with other herbs and is also a memory favorite of my patients.

(Always check herbs and supplements with your doctor if you
have a medical condition, including high blood pressure and
thyroid issues.)

Get a discount, if you are a new customer, when you mention
Dr. Lonsdorf's name to the representative or enter her name as
you establish your online account.

(Note: 100 percent of attributable commissions
go directly to charitable organizations for world peace and a
healthy planet.)

Call 1-800-255-8332 now or Register Online at *www.mapi.com*

6

Balance Your Hormones, Rejuvenate Your Brain

*There are three pillars of health—
diet, sleep, and balance of life.*

—Ayurveda aphorism

Key #6: Restore Optimal Hormone Levels

As a woman over 40, and possibly decades older, your brain may be aging faster than that of a man your age. Shocking news? Yes, indeed! In fact, this recent finding is the main reason this book is here now.

When I first learned of this research, I found it very disconcerting. I had spent the past two decades preaching the findings of the Women's Health Initiative, which concluded that risks of hormone replacement therapy (HRT) outweigh the benefits. I am also deeply committed to the wisdom of natural medicine, including Ayurveda, that philosophically holds that Nature "programmed" our bodies for good health. In this model, we ideally should be able to stay healthy in the face of "normal" transitions like menopause, without needing to take medicines.

Even now, I am convinced that Nature did not intend for us to deteriorate and wither up after menopause, but to live fully healthy, vital, and fulfilling lives for many more decades. In an ideal world, we would make enough hormones to keep our brains healthy, even after menopause. However, we don't live in an ideal world and healthy midlife brains are not what brain scans of peri- and post-menopausal women show today.

Neuroscientist Lisa Mosconi and colleagues recently found that women going through perimenopause and menopause show accelerated brain aging as compared to men of the same age. They evaluated a group of men and a group of women, matched in age (40 to 60) and scores on memory tests. They then performed two types of brain scans: PET scans to measure the levels of metabolism and amyloid level in their brains, and MRI scans to measure the size of specific brain regions.

In the younger subjects, around age 40, men and women were comparable on all measures. However, when comparing the measures between the sexes in those a bit older, around the age of perimenopause (45 to 50,) and then those past menopause age, the two groups diverged. After hormonal shifts set in, women's brain metabolism slowed down, an early sign of neuronal stress, amyloid deposition increased, and eventually greater volume loss (shrinkage) was seen in key memory and cognition areas of the brain. These brain changes appeared first in the perimenopausal years and continued to progress in the years following menopause.

These findings clearly implicate hormonal factors as an important contributor to women's 100 percent greater risk of Alzheimer's disease. Furthermore, they point the way toward potential preventive approaches. The researchers commented, "These data indicate that the optimal window of opportunity for therapeutic intervention in women is early in the endocrine aging process."

In other words, intervene early. Support a woman's brain during the times of often dramatic and erratic fluctuations at perimenopause, and also later, as growing estradiol deficiency sets in for most women. Give the brain the hormonal "trophic support" (growth factors) it needs to prevent, or at least slow, amyloid deposition that is occurring in the face of dropping estradiol levels. Midlife loss of estradiol, both a potent growth factor and an inhibitor of amyloid production in the brain, appears to set women up for a greater likelihood of cognitive decline later in life.

Clearly, we have a problem here. The question is, "what's a woman to do?" Does this mean every woman should take estrogen to prevent Alzheimer's? As usual, translating findings into practice with real women in the real world takes even more research to answer that question responsibly.

There are still many unanswered questions. For example, is perimenopause a true "window" of opportunity, meaning if you start HRT later, is it still helpful, or could it make things worse? Does HRT help when taken for only a few years around perimenopause, and is then stopped? Or must it be continued for a set period of time, or even throughout life? What is the optimal time to start, and perhaps to stop, HRT, to avoid cognitive decline down the line?

The questions surrounding hormone therapy seem to have become more complicated over time, not more clear-cut. However, one question has been settled quite confidently: bioidentical hormones (that exactly match the human body's own hormones) are associated with fewer side-effects than those used in the Women's Health Initiative.

In this chapter, I'll be referring to the form of hormone replacement therapy ideally prescribed to women today, as "BHRT," or bioidentical hormone replacement therapy. BHRT is now the recommended form of hormone replacement therapy due to its lower risk profile.

Thankfully, there are many approaches to supporting cognition and preventing Alzheimer's beyond taking hormones. At the end of this first section, I will describe many natural ways you can enhance and protect your memory and cognition if you prefer to avoid hormones, or taking hormones is not an option for you.

We'll delve into the details of these lifestyle approaches that can add joy to your life, support your vitality and fortify your brain with or without the additional support of HRT.

In order to understand the options available to you now, it'll be helpful to review how we got where we are today and the current status of the research on hormone therapy for perimenopausal and menopausal women.

Where We've Been—The Women's Health Initiative (WHI)

In the 1960s through the 1980s, doctors were prescribing hormone replacement therapy to prevent osteoporosis and heart disease, and also, because drug marketers had convinced women that it was a magical fountain of youth. Indeed, observational studies (i.e., surveys across a population) found that women who took HRT had less heart disease as well as less osteoporosis. But the question remained, was the cardiovascular benefit simply due to the fact that women who opted for hormones were simply more health conscious, and their healthier diet and lifestyle were the real causes of the reduction and heart disease.

The Women's Health Initiative (WHI) set out to answer that question. According to the NIH, the WHI, "is a long-term national health study that focuses on strategies for preventing heart disease, breast and colorectal cancer, and osteoporosis in postmenopausal women. ... The WHI was one of the most definitive, far-reaching clinical trials of post-menopausal women's health ever undertaken in the U.S."

Prior to the WHI, women had been excluded from many major clinical trials due to the perceived difficulty of controlling for monthly hormone fluctuations in premenopausal women and changing hormonal status with age. WHI was designed to rectify many of these inequities in women's health research.

One major aim of the WHI was to evaluate whether the benefits of hormone replacement therapy seen in prior observational studies would hold up in a randomized, double-blind controlled trial, the "gold standard" of clinical research. This clinical trial involved 16,608 healthy postmenopausal women aged 50 to 79 who were allocated to treatment with placebo or with 0.625 mg of conjugated equine estrogen ("CEE," from pregnant horses) and 2.5 mg of an artificial progesterone substitute, medroxyprogesterone acetate (MPA), required for those with a uterus.

What Caused the Dangerous Side-effects of the WHI?

The Type of Hormones Given—Not Bioidentical

First of all, the estrogen given in the WHI, Premarin, short for "pregnant mares urine," was collected from exactly that, pregnant female horses. The often inhumane conditions associated with such collection aside, Premarin contains at least 17 different forms of estrogen, all natural to a horse, but none an exact match for any of the three human forms of estrogen our bodies make: estradiol (the most potent one, plentiful in the brain), estriol (least potent, highest during pregnancy), and estrone (the most plentiful estrogen in the body after menopause).

In addition, medroxyprogesterone, the artificial "progestin" given in the WHI to protect the uterus from cancer caused by giving estrogen alone, is not a match for our own "progesterone" molecule but is a roughly related chemical synthesized in a laboratory. This artificial progestin, evidence suggests, was the real culprit for much of the negative impact of HRT revealed by the WHI, considerably more than estrogen itself.

It is critical to keep in mind that all WHI findings resulted from these non-human, non-bioidentical hormones. Neither matched the estrogen and progesterone that our own bodies make. That poses a recipe for imbalances, as these chemicals do not interact with our body in the same way that our own hormones do. They are not an exact "fit" for our hormone receptors, which bind the hormone and trigger a response inside each cell. The response triggered will be different because the molecule interacts with the receptor differently than our own hormones do. It's rather like trying to open a lock using a slightly misshapen key. It doesn't work smoothly.

Estrogen Given Orally

Another contributor to side-effects in the WHI was orally administered estrogen. We now know that oral administration of estrogen results in excess clotting as the hormones pass through the liver, increasing a multitude of clotting factors, before they continue on to the rest of the body. This can increase blood clots in the legs or the lungs, as well as promote strokes and heart attacks.

To avoid these complications, bioidentical estrogens today are commonly prescribed in the form of a transdermal patch, (estrogen enters the body through the skin,) or vaginally.

Early Termination of the Women's Health Initiative

In 2002, the WHI grabbed global headlines when it was terminated early due to the overall assessment that the side effects of HRT, including increased breast cancer risk, heart attacks, strokes, blood clots, dementia, and gallbladder disease, to name a few, exceeded the benefits. The early termination of the WHI rocked the medical community and a whole generation of women over forty. Prescriptions of HRT fell precipitously as doctors and patients alike decided that symptoms of menopause were preferable to increased heart disease and cancer risk.

What went wrong? Here's a bottom-line summary of how the specific type of HRT in the WHI created so many detrimental effects:

- Women were given non-bioidentical horse estrogen and "progestin" from a lab, not a woman's body's own forms of estrogen and progesterone.
- Artificial "progestin" use was associated with increased heart disease and breast cancer, whereas the horse estrogen alone was not.
- The horse estrogen was given by mouth, which increases clotting via the "first pass liver effect," resulting in more strokes, including in those women taking estrogen alone, without the artificial progestin.
- Increase in breast cancer was seen only in the women taking the artificial progestin, not in the women taking horse estrogen alone. In those taking horse estrogen alone, breast cancer incidence was actually reduced.
- "Probable dementia" doubled in those women over 65 who were given both horse estrogen and progestin. Those on horse estrogen alone had no increase and possibly a reduction in dementia risk.
- Younger women, in their 50s, generally had fewer side effects, including no increase in heart disease risk with or without progestin, and no negative effect on cognition. In fact, they showed a reduction in cardiovascular disease while on HRT.

Fast Forward: Bioidentical Hormone Replacement Therapy (BHRT)

Today it's a "whole new world" in the hormone arena. Since 2002, a growing number of studies have set out to evaluate the effects of a very different approach to hormone therapy, termed "bioidentical hormone replacement therapy," or BHRT. BHRT uses hormones that are exact replicas of a woman's own and seeks to administer it in a way that minimizes side-effects.

A lot has been learned about hormone metabolism and safety since the WHI. Here's a short list of important features to keep in mind:

- BHRT hormones exactly match a woman's own hormone structures.
- Estrogens are administered through the skin or vaginally, not by mouth, to avoid increased clotting risk.
- Progesterone is "bioidentical," and can be given by mouth or vaginally. Progesterone must be given to all women with a uterus who are taking estrogen to prevent uterine cancer.

So far, research on BHRT has yielded a different, generally more positive, spectrum of results as compared to the WHI. This could be expected, as they use very different formulations and routes of administration. While an exhaustive review is beyond the scope of this book, let's look at the most pertinent research highlights that can help you decide if you want to take BHRT or not.

- Beneficial effects on cognition were found in 15 of 17 studies using transdermal estradiol via a "patch," gel or cream, according to a review by Wharton et al.
- A greater number of years on estrogen is associated with healthier brain metabolism, including the hippocampus and other Alzheimer's-prone brain regions, according to a study by Silverman et al.
- Silverman also found bioidentical estradiol use resulted in markedly better verbal memory performance than the use of horse estrogen (CEE).

- Estradiol use lowered the risk of heart disease, stroke, and all causes of death very significantly if used for at least 10 years. No difference in effect was found if started before age 60 versus after in this study by Mikkola et al.
- Only one study, the KEEPS trial, looked at breast cancer risk with transdermal estradiol plus bioidentical progesterone. Over 4 years, no increase in breast cancer was noted.

Will Taking Estrogen Help Your Memory?

So far, the evidence indicates that taking bioidentical estrogen in the form of estradiol may help your memory later in life, and help you avoid all-out dementia, as long as you do not take the artificial progestin, MPA, along with it. There's no evidence to date that it will help with your "senior moments," name-finding, or other age-related memory slip-ups, but we're certainly open to that possibility!

You may recall from Chapter One, that there is a subset of women with memory loss and cognitive decline that is caused by toxic exposure, referred to as "type 3" Alzheimer's disease. Clinical experience indicates that women with the type 3, "toxic" form in particular benefit from optimizing their hormones.

It is not unusual for these women to date the onset of their cognitive issues to perimenopause or menopause and, as such, may be particularly well-positioned to get more benefit than risk from taking bioidentical hormones. If you feel this applies to you, be sure to discuss BHRT with your doctor.

Bioidentical hormones are available, by the way, through most conventional doctors in the form of estradiol (usually offered in a transdermal patch form) and oral progesterone, called "Prometrium." While maximal recovery will require more than just fixing hormones, you may recall that Dr. Bredesen's Patient Zero

"Kristin," felt that restarting her hormones was a key factor in her nearly miraculous, complete cognitive comeback.

Bioidentical hormone therapy may in the end prove to be a "necessary, though not sufficient" factor that your optimal memory function, or recovery thereof, may require—or not. Obviously, this is a decision you need to make with your doctor, who will ideally be conversant with the latest literature and "consensus" opinions from the North American Menopause Society and other medical institutions.

Is There an Optimal "Window of Opportunity?"

Evidence points to the benefits of starting BHRT early, for example during perimenopause, and continuing for at least several years after menstruation completely ceases. Research indicates that side-effects are usually fewer in this younger age group but may increase to the point of adverse effects on cognition if begun too late in life, such as after 65 or 70 years old, particularly with non-bioidentical estrogen and artificial progestin.

On the other hand, further research points to a very interesting possibility. Women of any age who score in an average to above-average level on cognitive testing may stand to benefit later in life from taking BHRT. It may actually be that healthy neurons nourished with estradiol help women maintain their normal function, growth, and connections. If neurons are already degenerating, such as in women with failing cognition, giving hormones may have adverse effects.

Researchers have postulated that changes in how estradiol influences regulation of genes and mitochondrial function may lie at the heart of this age-related discrepancy, which may eventually bear out to be due more to your brain's "biological age" than to chronological age. (Biological age means how healthy and youthful your neurons are, regardless of your age in years.)

This opens the possibility for women over 65 to start and potentially benefit cognitively from BHRT if your cognition is currently in a good place. Formal memory and cognitive testing can help assess that. Obviously, this is a complex decision, and all the data isn't in yet. You'll need to consult with your doctor to determine what is right for you.*

Is There An Age You Should Stop BHRT?

So far, there is no definitive reason to stop BHRT simply due to age. In fact, Mikkola et al. found that the longer you take BHRT, the greater the benefits. Taking BHRT resulted in a drop in all causes of death by a range of 12 to 38 percent, almost in direct proportion to how many years it was taken. Also, results were comparable in women who started BHRT before age 60 versus after age 60. Not all studies bear that out. However, their finding is encouraging for menopausal women of all ages and may open the door for further studies on BHRT to definitively answer this question.

Do You Need Testosterone?

The short answer is, "not for cognition." Even in men, with low or with normal testosterone levels, supplementation has given variable results in studies to date. The data is not as clear as for estradiol in women. Testosterone can increase libido in some women and possibly have other benefits. Generally, testosterone can unfavorably affect your lipid profile, and should be considered as a separate issue, not automatically included in BHRT.

---

* Refer to the MoCA test described in Chapter One. In addition, your doctor may be able to give you access to the more in-depth CNS Vital Signs testing online or in her office. This computerized assessment tool is more detailed than the MoCA and can help identify more subtle degrees of impairment in defined areas of cognitive function.

Should You Still Be Concerned About Breast Cancer from BHRT?

There is very limited evidence to answer this question. In the WHI, only women taking MPA (artificial progestin) had an increase incidence. Those taking only the estrogen did not show increased risk and some analyses show they had lower risk than women on placebo.

The KEEPS Trial is the only one to date that looked at BHRT and breast cancer risk. In a 4-year follow-up of women taking either transdermal estradiol or CEE (horse estrogen) plus bioidentical progesterone, no increase in breast cancer incidence was found.

Does that mean you shouldn't be concerned about the possibility of breast cancer from BHRT? The evidence is too limited to answer that scientifically. It is a question for you to discuss with your doctor. If you have had an estrogen-receptor positive breast cancer, you may have extra concern about taking estradiol and been told by your oncologist never, ever to take estrogen or anything potentially estrogenic.

A number of physicians specializing in BHRT have reported (in as yet unpublished data) they have safely given estradiol to dozens of women who had ER+ (estrogen receptor-positive) breast cancer who were suffering from severe estrogen-deficiency symptoms and have not seen cancer recurrences in these patients.

More research is desperately needed on this issue. Unfortunately, it is unlikely to happen as long as the dogma prevails that estrogens must in all cases be avoided forever following a diagnosis of estrogen-receptor positive breast cancer. I'm not saying this is right or wrong, just that post-menopausal breast cancer survivors who are suffering from estrogen deprivation symptoms deserve an answer backed by actual data from clinical trials, rather than theory alone.

Does Estriol (E3) Protect the Brain?

The short answer is, "the brain likes estradiol (E2) best!" Estriol has not been shown to have a protective effect on cognition. Rather, estriol is great for vaginal tissue, and thankfully does not tend to overstimulate the uterine lining (meaning it is less likely to provoke uterine cancer than estradiol).

In the brain, however, the predominant type of estrogen receptor and the beneficial effects on cognition come from estradiol, not estriol. This means, the brain is "wired" to bind and respond to the estradiol (E2) form of estrogen, and research verifies its powerful positive, trophic (growth-promoting) effect on brain tissue.

What Should You Do Next? Check Your Hormone Levels!

Let's get back to the optimal values that Dr. Bredesen and his team have used to guide their work in reversing cognitive decline. The optimal minimum value for estradiol is set at 50, though some doctors hold that 30 to 50 is enough for some women.

To put these values in perspective, I have found estradiol levels ranging from "less than 5" all the way up to 39 in post-menopausal women who are not taking any hormones. This shows that women vary a lot in how much their bodies are producing on their own. Generally, women with low body fat tend to have lower estradiol levels. However, the best way to assess yourself is to get your hormone levels tested with a simple blood test. If your level is close to or above 30, you may want to accept that as enough.

Also, you may want to check with a specialist to see if your body is making enough progesterone to balance your relatively plentiful estradiol. If not, this "estrogen dominance" can put you at increased risk of uterine cancer, in which case bioidentical progesterone, vaginally or orally, might be beneficial to you.

Note: Ask your doctor for a prescription for oral or vaginal progesterone, rather than reaching for over-the-counter topical progesterone creams. Progesterone is highly fat soluble and when applied regularly through the skin, can lead to very high levels in body tissues (as shown by saliva and capillary blood levels, though not always on blood tests).

If your estradiol is very low, you may want to see your gynecologist or a BHRT specialist (who may or may not be as objective) to discuss whether BHRT is right for you.

Go to *www.thehealthybrainsolution.com* for a list of online options for hormone blood testing—as well as a sample order you can take to your doctor.

Where I Stand...

I have been cautious about prescribing hormone therapy for over 20 years, having seen numerous side-effects in my mother's generation on WHI-type hormones. I also possess a "Nature knows best" bias in favor of creating balance without drugs or hormones whenever possible. Finally, my heartfelt commitment to the Hippocratic injunction, "First, do no harm," has led to my continued reluctance to prescribe hormones when there is no immediate suffering at hand.

Hearing about, studying, and pondering the growing evidence on the relative safety and potential benefits of BHRT has certainly begun to "turn my head around" on the issue, and I do believe it has a role in preventing cognitive decline in select, and possibly many or even most women.

At the same time, I believe we should do all we can to optimize our hormones, our health, and our cognition through diet and lifestyle, the inescapable foundation of our health. As one of my favorite Ayurvedic adages goes "Without proper diet (and lifestyle), medicines are of no use. With proper diet, medicines are of no need!"

According to menopause expert and founding director of the North American Menopause Society, Dr. Utian Wulf, the solution to the hormone dilemma is not "one size fits all," and may well be different for each woman. In Change Your Menopause, Dr. Wulf reviews research on the pros and cons of bioidentical hormone therapy and outlines a highly individualized approach that incorporates non-hormonal diet, lifestyle, and supplement programs tailored to the needs and preferences of each woman.

In the next section, I'll address how to optimize your hormones by supporting your adrenal glands, a primary source of hormones after menopause, through stress reduction, sleep, eating habits, exercise, and the optimal daily schedule for all of these.

Natural Approach To Hormone Balancing

It is not necessary for everyone to take hormones for prevention, especially if you don't have cognitive decline, hot flashes, or any other symptoms. In every case, I recommend women incorporate the natural approach that Ayurveda prescribes with herbs, diet, and proper lifestyle based on your type or dosha—regardless of your chosen interventions. Ayurveda provides a unique angle on healing that no other approach can replace.

According to Ayurveda, two of the best herbs for women are shatavari (Asparagus racemosus) and ashwagandha. Shatavari has been shown to attach to estradiol receptors and is demonstrated to have pro-estrogenic effects. However, as with most plant-based estrogens, shatavari's action is not one-dimensional as drugs tend to be, but more complex, with balance being the rule.

For example, while shatavari may stimulate certain estradiol receptors, it has also been shown to inhibit other estrogen receptors, potentially lowering breast cancer risk. Shatavari also helps

165

curb heavy menstrual bleeding, commonly attributable to excess estrogen.

From an Ayurvedic perspective, shatavari is both vata- and pitta-pacifying (i.e., calming and cooling). Available in tablet form, you can start with one tablet (500 mg) twice a day. You may take up to two tablets twice a day, if needed, for greater effects.

Ashwagandha is an "adaptogen" herb, (meaning it helps the body cope with stress,) that has also been shown to directly inhibit amyloid production and support neuron regeneration and healing. It is very vata-balancing (calming and strengthening for nerves and hormones) for both women and men.

For low testosterone levels in women, I usually recommend measures that promote optimal testosterone levels, or mimic its effects, rather than taking testosterone hormone replacement. Simply getting enough sleep, reducing stress, and eating wholesome, balanced food on a regular schedule can help normalize your adrenal function and support testosterone production.

Herbal supplements such as ashwagandha, maca root and tribulus terrestris may all be helpful in supporting libido and sexual function, the primary reason most women request testosterone supplementation, in my experience. Beware of chronic mental, emotional, and physical stress as all can lower your testosterone levels. Especially in the case of women, addressing the root causes of testosterone deficiency will accomplish more for your long-term health than taking the hormone as a supplement.

Testing Method: Adrenal Glands

Your adrenal glands play a key role in your hormone balance. Located atop each kidney, the adrenal glands produce several hormones vital to life, such as cortisol, our stress-handling hormone, and aldosterone, which helps maintain proper fluid balance in the body. Our adrenals also provide a backup source for our reproductive hormones estrogen, progesterone, and testosterone.

After menopause, as ovarian estrogen production dramatically drops, adrenal sex hormone production is especially important. Excess stress, however, can "steal" the adrenals' limited supply of hormone building blocks in favor of making life-essential cortisol, rather than our more expendable sex hormones and rejuvenative hormones such as DHEA.

In this way, chronic stress can lead to excess cortisol and abnormally low estrogen levels after menopause, along with collagen loss (think sagging skin), bone loss (osteoporosis), and potentially, excessive brain shrinkage. Moreover, excess cortisol has been implicated in sleep disturbance as well as type 2 diabetes, obesity, and cardiovascular disease, all brain-busters in their own right.

Ellen's Story—An Undiagnosed Hormone Excess

Ellen is a newly retired, 58-year-old corporate executive who came to me complaining of constant worry and insomnia. She had made a good living and had comfortable savings, so money was not an issue. She was happy with her new life and in good physical condition. She was perplexed as to why she was worrying all the time and suddenly couldn't sleep at night. What was causing this distress?

I saw on her intake form that Ellen had been taking bioidentical hormone therapy (BHRT) for several years, in the form of rub-on creams for both estradiol and progesterone. She said the hormones had helped her around the time of her menopause, as she had suffered "brain fog" and embarrassing memory lapses that were not compatible with her usual high performance and what she, and others, expected of her in her leadership position. She assured me that the prescribing doctor was monitoring her blood levels and they were always in line.

However, her prescribing physician was apparently unaware of the "partitioning" of hormones, particularly of highly fat-soluble progesterone, which can result in very different levels in serum versus blood spot (capillary blood from a fingerstick) or saliva levels. When progesterone is administered through the skin, it is more accurately measured through blood spot or saliva samples—rather than the conventional blood test Ellen's doctor used—according to research by David Zava, PhD, and colleagues, who directly tackled this thorny controversial issue with objective studies.

In Ellen's case, I recommended a saliva test to check her hormone levels, including her stress hormone, cortisol, which, as a member of the same "steroid hormone family" can interconvert with progesterone. Indeed, Ellen's test results showed her estradiol and progesterone levels were both very high, as was her cortisol, the latter most likely due to conversion of excess progesterone into cortisol.

Ellen's extremely high cortisol levels had sent her body inadvertently into a constant fight or flight mode. In a sense, her usual calm and focused mind and brain were hijacked by a raging hormonal storm. Fortunately, with a major reduction in hormone dosage, Ellen's anxiety and insomnia gradually abated, restoring her peace of mind and usual sound sleep within a few months.

Ellen's story is not unique. Sarah, a patient of about the same age, had a similar story. She had been put on BHRT creams during her perimenopause, about 5 years before. She came to me due to steadily worsening insomnia and depression, which she had never before experienced in her life. As a strong "executive type," her newfound feelings of anxiety, insomnia, and depression baffled her. She found it very discouraging and frustrating to have to take both a sleeping pill and an anti-depressant just to function each day. "I'm not a depressive person," she lamented.

Upon testing, Sarah's saliva hormone panel revealed a similar pattern as Ellen's—an elevated cortisol and very high levels of progesterone, over 2000 (normal is 500 or less.) It took about a year for Sarah's hormones to return to normal—on a much lower progesterone dose given orally—and another 6 months to slowly taper off her medications. Finally, she was able to sleep again, recovered fully from her depression and had no need for medication.

I bring up these stories to highlight that both of these women's symptoms stemmed from progesterone applied as a topical cream—a highly popularized, over-the-counter approach in the 1990s and early 2000s. Even today, topical progesterone is available without a prescription, as an over-the-counter preparation. My advice is simple: buyer beware. Don't take progesterone as a topical skin cream unless your doctor is also monitoring your levels by saliva or blood spot testing.

One more word of caution, always carefully read the labels on your skin care products. Unfortunately, many products have added hormones, such as DHEA, in amounts not specified and perhaps not carefully controlled. Unsuspectingly ingesting these compounds can play havoc with your body's delicate hormonal balance and create symptoms that you may never otherwise know the source of.

Rest and Exercise / Restore and Strengthen

Research shows that maintaining balanced hormones, reducing stress levels, properly nourishing your body and brain, and getting your blood pumping through exercise can go a long way toward keeping your brain healthy and your memory vital for a lifetime. Let's take a closer look at how our lifestyle can benefit our brains and identify the most important actions to adopt and maintain over time.

Cycles of Rest and Activity

Sleep, diet, and balance of life are the three pillars of health, according to the texts of Ayurveda. Ayurvedic rishis ("seers" credited with directly cognizing or intuiting the laws of Nature governing health) deeply understood the principles of healing with regard to diet, herbs, and lifestyle. Somehow, they knew that our bodies follow a rhythmic 24-hour cycle of metabolic, hormonal, and physiological activity, and that our health depends on aligning our daily routine to match Nature's inner and outer rhythms.

As the earth turns on its axis, rotating us toward or away from the warm, nourishing rays of the sun, our bodies respond with corresponding 24-hour rhythms that cue us to the optimal time of day to eat our biggest meal, go to bed, get up in the morning, and exercise.

When our outer daily schedule aligns with our body's inner biorhythm, we feel our best, digest optimally, optimize our cardiovascular health and immunity, and move through the day with least effort and stress. Even before modern research came to validate this ancient principle, my patients frequently reported how much the recommended Ayurvedic schedule "resonated" with them, "made sense," and bestowed many benefits.

After 30 years of rewarding clinical results, I have been delighted to discover the growing body of pioneering research in chronobiology (the science of how time affects our bodies) that supports many of the Ayurvedic prescriptions for "what to do when."

"In-Sync" for Better Sleep

I recently took an informal poll of 15 to 20 people, about half of whom described themselves as "night owls" and half as "morning larks." Inquiring further into how well they felt they slept at night, nearly every one of the "morning larks," who go to bed early, slept well, and less than half of the "night owls" claimed good sleep. Informal research as it is, it reflects what I commonly see in my practice.

One of my patients, a woman several years past menopause, wrote me to say that she had slept poorly for years and simply resigned herself to the idea that "this was menopause," and she'd probably never sleep well again.

The day I told her of the benefits of going to bed early, she returned from a business trip and, instead of her usual compulsive unpacking late into the night, she turned in early, by 10 p.m. Guess what? In her words, she "slept like a baby." That hadn't happened for years!

Likewise, an obstetrician-gynecologist colleague of mine had difficulty sleeping through the night after years of middle-of-the-night deliveries and two babies of her own. One year, her husband took up ocean sailing, taking her and their children along, and spending many days at sea between dockings.

"I've never sleep as well as I do on the boat," she recounts. "There's no TV, no internet, or cell phone. We eat dinner and then hang out enjoying the sea, the sunset, and each other. Everyone starts to feel tired at 8:30 or so, just as it's getting dark, and with nothing else to do, we all go to bed. Amazingly, I sleep deeply and wake up refreshed. It all feels so natural. It's hard to believe something as simple as sleep could have become so difficult. It's really meant to be easy and effortless."

There are many more everyday examples of the wonders of an aligned daily schedule, but let's look at the research.

In short, there are three key Ayurvedic schedule recommendations for good health:

- Go to sleep by 10 p.m.
- Eat your main meal by noon or 1 p.m.
- Exercise between 6 and 10 in the morning or evening.

Calling All Performers!

One musician wrote me about his professional inability to go to bed early, obviously a bit upset that there didn't seem to be a place for his typical schedule in an "Ayurvedically kosher" lifestyle. He commented: "I find my body has found its own rhythm and it's not what you are recommending. Nor can any other performer follow your prescription. ... Only by following my instinct and training (i.e., making peace and going with the flow of a late bedtime after performances) have I been happy and prosperous."

While I firmly believe, and research verifies that we are "day creatures," with our cellular and master brain "clocks" resetting each day by the rising sun, I also believe the human body has a tremendous ability to adapt itself to changing circumstances, especially when they are regularly maintained. An irregular routine, on the other hand, as with variable shift work, is the hardest on our bodies, per the research.

I find the musician's comment that "my body has found its own rhythm" says it all. Ayurveda is not dogma. It does point out the natural, optimal direction, but our bodies will also adapt the best they can to whatever schedule we choose to keep.

In my experience, individuals vary a lot in their ability to withstand a nighttime or variable awake schedule, with age and personal constitution both playing a role. While more innately stressful than naturally rising and retiring with the sun, performers' schedules just do not follow the usual laws of Nature, so over time, the body thankfully adjusts.

The Power of a Good Night's Sleep

We don't need medical research to know that sleep matters for our health and our brains. We all have noticed how much better we feel and perform, when we have had a good night's sleep.

Mounting evidence indeed points to a connection between sleep quantity and cognitive function. When we don't get enough sleep, our ability to recall details is impaired as is reaction time and our ability to think clearly. Problem-solving ability also suffers. Poor sleep raises levels of cortisol, the stress hormone, weakens the immune system, and sadly, accelerates aging.

Most Americans are sleep deprived. In their first study of self-reported sleep length, the U.S. Centers for Disease Control and Prevention found that 34.8 percent of American adults are getting less than 7 hours of sleep—the minimum length of time adults should sleep in order to reduce risk of obesity, diabetes, high blood pressure, stroke, mental distress, coronary heart disease, and early death.

Many of my women patients over 40 complain of waking up in the middle of the night for a few hours. When this happens, they find themselves dragging through the next day, resorting to caffeine to keep going, which may in turn, disturb their next night's sleep. If this routine happens frequently, they are seriously sleep deprived.

Besides the usual health risks, type 2 diabetes, obesity, and cardiovascular disease, inadequate sleep increases irritability, mood swings, stressful feelings, and is a known risk factor for cognitive decline. In fact, insomnia is such a strong risk factor for cognitive decline that many long-term care insurers will disqualify applicants who list insomnia or sleep disturbance as one of their health issues, as well as, of course, memory issues. On the practical side, take note of this if you are considering applying for such insurance.

Oxygen and Your Sleep

Are you breathing well at night? Even if you've slept enough hours, if you're not breathing well, you may wake up feeling tired or may experience drowsiness during quieter moments of the day—such as that boring committee meeting or lecture! I advise all my Healthy Brain Program patients to order and perform a home test for sleep apnea. Inexpensive and available online (and now increasingly available through your local doctor or hospital), these simple do-at-home devices are comfortable to wear and give a reliable measure of hypoxia (low blood oxygen) that can signal airway blockage during the night.

If you snore, or your partner notices you stop breathing or have sudden deep breaths in the night, or you feel tired or fall asleep easily during the day despite enough sleep, I urge you to take such a test. If it's normal, you can forget about it as an issue, as long as you don't develop new symptoms. If it's not normal, see your doctor for a discussion of options.

Upper airway blockage (UARS) is especially common in women and can be easier to treat than lower airway obstruction. Sometimes a simple dental appliance is all it takes to keep the back of the throat open, with no need for a bulky CPAP device. In any case, get yourself checked and do what it takes to breathe properly at night—it's critical to your memory and future brain health.

Our Sleep After 40

Menopausal symptoms and hormonal imbalance, such as low progesterone, as well as depression and stress are frequent contributors to sleep problems in midlife women. Correcting these issues, with or without hormones, is often helpful.

In addition, I've observed that dysbiosis, or indigestion, may play a role sleep disturbance in some women. Taking a good probiotic, such as the spore-based one discussed in Chapter Two, may be helpful, as well as seeing a functional medicine doctor for a more thorough microbiome evaluation, i.e. presence of any parasites, yeast, or dysbiotic flora.

The Ketoflex 12/3 routine of avoiding eating for 3 hours before bed also promotes better sleep by preventing insulin secretion, which inhibits melatonin and growth hormone. The Ayurvedic recommendation is to avoid meat, cheese, and other hard-to-digest, "heavy" foods in the evening.

Reassuringly, as much as good sleep is considered essential to a cognitive recovery program, a monumental review study by Scullin and Bliwise, integrating research across multiple disciplines over 50 years, showed that lower quality sleep as we get older may not be as detrimental as we've thought. Rather, poor sleep may impair cognition more in young and midlife people, as measured by their cognitive function for age, a predictor of later decline.

So, if your sleep isn't great, keep working on improving it, but stop worrying. Maybe you'll even sleep better as a result! (Indeed, cognitive therapy focused on reducing anxiety about not sleeping has been shown to improve both sleep time and quality.)

As we've touched on before, research has uncovered the amazing fact that a key function of sleep is to clean the cells of your brain. While our brains sleep, harmful toxins such as metabolic wastes and even amyloid can be removed by our innate "housekeeping" functions, including autophagy. Obviously, enhancing that process through good sleep and induction of a ketotic metabolic state (via the 12/3 eating routine,) is in our memory's best interest!

The Data on Early Bedtime

In a U.S. National Longitudinal Study of Adolescent Health, researchers compared students randomized to a bedtime of 10 p.m. versus midnight. The results showed students staying up until midnight were 24 percent more likely to be depressed, and 20 percent more likely to have suicidal thoughts.

A further study showed that the benefits of going to bed early were not a result of getting more sleep. In addition, the effects were long-lasting: those going to bed before 11:15 p.m. in high school had better academic achievement and less emotional distress when followed up as long as 6 years later. According to Ayurveda, and accumulating research, early to bed is key to better sleep, a more positive mood, and being your cognitive best for the next day's activities.

Tips for a Good Night's Sleep

- Keep a consistent sleep schedule, ideally going to bed by 10 p.m. Get up at the same time every day (ideal is by 6 a.m.), even on weekends or during vacations.
- Make your bedroom quiet and relaxing. Turn off your Wi-Fi at night, if you can, and all electronic devices, including TV and iPhone at least 30 minutes before bedtime. Keep the TV out of your bedroom.
- Keep your bedroom at a comfortable, cool temperature and block light from the windows as much as possible.
- Do not work in your bedroom, if at all possible. Use your bedroom for sleep.
- Establish a relaxing bedtime routine. Avoid vigorous exercise too close to bedtime. Instead, take a brief leisurely walk followed by a relaxing bath when you can.
- Limit exposure to bright light in the evenings and cut blue light at night. Get one of the popular apps now available that promise better sleep by filtering out the blue light produced by iPhones, tablets, computers, and even televisions. Alternatively, try "blue blocker" orange-tinted glasses in the evening.
- Your brain naturally produces melatonin at night but only if it is dark. If you are exposed to light, especially blue light, in the evening, melatonin production is inhibited. As mel-

atonin production tends to decline with age, many people get better sleep by taking 0.5 mg to 1 mg of melatonin at bedtime. This lower dose is recommended by many integrative physicians, rather than the more common high dose pills, as the lower dose more closely approximates your body's own production.

- Avoid consuming caffeine in the late afternoon or evening.
- Avoid drinking alcohol before bedtime. While alcohol can help some women feel sleepy, it is toxic to neurons, interferes with sleeping through the night, and can trigger more hot flashes.
- Reduce your fluid intake before bedtime so that you don't awake in the middle of the night for a bathroom run.
- Eat your dinner by 7 p.m. at the latest. Eating early improves sleep and also helps prevent joint pains and sinus congestion. Eat a light, easy-to-digest meal for dinner.
- Don't eat for 3 hours before going to bed. A reminder: this short period of fasting will start the brain's housecleaning, in the natural process called autophagy (literally "self-eating"), the body's built-in system for cleaning house. Your cells create membranous vesicles called autophagosomes that seek out dead, diseased, or worn-out cell parts and metabolic wastes. They gobble them up, strip them for parts, and use the resulting molecules for energy or to make new cell parts. Our own internal recycling system!
- At bedtime, you may want to apply a little coconut oil to your scalp and/or the bottom of your feet. Amazingly, this simple practice can calm your nerves and help you settle down to sleep. Rub the coconut oil in your hands to melt it, then slip the palm of your hand underneath your hair to apply directly to your scalp. Massaging oil into scalp and the soles of your feet at bedtime can be sur-

prisingly relaxing and a fast-acting cure for sleep-busting "monkey-mind."

Dinner at Noon—Like Those Close To the Land

When I was a kid, my classmates living on farms used to call lunch "dinner," and their evening meal "supper." Now I understand why. Being in tune with the land and Nature, their families traditionally ate their main meal, "dinner," in the middle of the day, when the body can best process and use a major intake of nutrition.

In practice, I find that eating the main meal at lunchtime helps prevent late afternoon "munchies," and allows you to eat a lighter evening meal, better for sound sleep, autophagy, and rejuvenation of the brain and whole body during the night. Patients also tell me they no longer arrive home starving and can avoid devouring everything in sight before they get dinner prepared and on the table.

Another side benefit of eating your main meal at noon is better metabolism and weight management, even while consuming the same number of calories. A study of 420 subjects published in the International Journal of Obesity (3) showed that those randomized to eating the majority of their calories before 3 p.m. had more and quicker weight loss than those eating the majority of their calories after 3 p.m.—even though they consumed the same number of total calories. The researchers concluded that "novel approaches" to weight loss that include the timing of meals should be considered in any weight loss program.

Research in progress at the Salk Institute recently found that restricting eating to a 10-hour period during the day (i.e., fasting at least 14 consecutive hours out of every 24-hour cycle) significantly improved sleep duration and quality, as well as blood sugar control. Chalk up one more benefit of "intermittent fasting" (going at least 12 hours without eating in each 24-hour period)—better sleep!

The Gifts of Exercise

There are two main points worth knowing about exercise and your brain.

First of all, all three major forms of exercise—continuous aerobic (steady pace), high-intensity interval training or "HIIT" (alternating fast and slow aerobic), and resistance training (lifting weights, etc.) are effective, with each yielding its own respective profile of benefits.

In one recent comparison study, Coetsee and Terblanche found that resistance training and continuous aerobic activity resulted in greatest gains for executive function (attention, planning, and self-regulation tasks) while high-intensity interval training resulted in greater physical endurance as well as faster brain processing speed. (Interesting that practicing intervals of "all out, as fast as you can" sprinting translates into ever faster "fast as you can" brain speed!)

The authors conclude that more studies should be done on exercise and cognition, especially regarding high-intensity interval training alone or in combination with other exercise modalities, and with a wider variety of cognitive measures.

Better oxygenation, increased blood flow, stimulation of new neurons and synapses, as well as the hormones that regulate them such as BDNF (brain-derived neurotrophic factor) and IGF-1 have all been cited and demonstrated to play a role in the many cognitive benefits of exercise.

What is High-Intensity Interval Training (HIIT)?

HIIT is a training technique of giving all-out, 100 percent effort with quick, intense bursts of exercise, followed by slower recovery periods. A commonly recommended ratio is 1 part fast, "all out" exercise, followed by 3 parts slower, relaxed pace. Examples could be 15 seconds fast, 45 seconds slow; or 30 seconds fast, 90 seconds slow, for example. The sequence is then repeated over and over again for about 20 minutes.

Do consult your doctor before beginning a new exercise routine, if you have a medical condition, or haven't exercised regularly in some time. Now, here's a suggested workout that follows HIIT principles: After warming up for several minutes at an easy pace, exercise as fast as you can on a treadmill, elliptical, or sidewalk, for 15 seconds, then take it easy and recover for 45 seconds, moving at a much slower pace. Repeat this cycle several times, starting with as little as 5 total minutes and building up gradually as your level of endurance grows, and it will!

Exercise—How Much?

Fortunately, we now have a simple answer to this question. Researchers Joyce Gomes-Osman et al. surveyed 98 different studies on exercise and cognition. What they found is very straightforward: cognitive improvements occurred across all exercise types and timings when participants exercised at least 52 hours over a 6-month period. That means about 2 hours per week on average.

The number of minutes in each exercise session, the number of minutes exercising each week and the frequency of sessions were not significant factors—only the total exercise hours over the 6-month period mattered.

In their review, cognitive benefits were associated with all three types of exercise—aerobic, resistance/strength training, and "mind-body" exercises such as yoga—in the areas of global cognitive functioning, executive functioning and processing speed/attention.

Dr. Gomes-Osman commented that improvements in brain processing speed and executive functioning as a result of exercise, "is an encouraging result, because those two constructs are among the first that start to go with the aging process. This is evidence that you can actually turn back the clock of aging in your brain by adopting a regular exercise regimen," encouraging news indeed!

Exercise—The When

We know we should exercise, but when best to fit it in? First of all, I like to tell my patients that with today's overly busy schedules, exercise anytime is better than not at all. But beyond that, there are optimal times to exercise in the daily cycle.

Ayurveda recommends exercising in the "kapha time," between 6 and 10 in the morning or evening—with the morning being ideal. During these times, the body tends to be more stable, resilient, and possibly a bit sluggish. This is when you will benefit the most from physical activity, with the least likelihood of strain or injury.

A fascinating study on people with early hypertension bears this Ayurvedic recommendation out. Researchers looked at the blood pressure drop during sleep in relation to what time of day the subjects did aerobic exercise—either 7 a.m., 1 p.m., or 7 p.m. Normally, blood pressure drops during our sleep, with a greater drop predictive of better heart health and less likelihood of progressing from pre-hypertension to hypertension.

In line with the Ayurvedic prediction, morning exercise at 7 a.m. resulted in the greatest nighttime drop in systolic blood pressure, as well as the added bonus of deeper sleep. Second place went to exercising at 7 p.m., which resulted in the greatest drop in diastolic nocturnal blood pressure.

On the other hand, those who exercised at 1 p.m., lunchtime, actually showed barely any nighttime drop in blood pressure, rather there was inhibition of the desired effect. True to the Ayurvedic maxim, "after lunch, rest awhile, after dinner, walk a mile," it's better to eat, rest, and digest at lunchtime, and leave your workout to earlier or later in the day.

This finding allowed me a bit of personal redemption, beyond the validation of an Ayurvedic principle. When I was in my psychiatry residency, I used to meditate at lunchtime rather than join my colleagues in their sweaty midday jog around the VA grounds in the hot, California sun. Now I see I may have had the healthier instinct!

The *Real* Power Walk

In ancient times, the great Ayurvedic physician, Charak, was teaching in a forest amphitheater, with his disciples gathered in a circle around him. One of them asked the great master, "Is there anything that balances the entire mind and body, promotes elimination, increases immunity and inner purity, and is suitable for all ages, can be done in all seasons everywhere in the world, and does not cost anything?" The great sage answered, "Yes, wake up early in the morning and take a walk in the light of the rising sun."

Ayurveda has always recommended a morning walk as the best overall rejuvenating and healthy habit we can adopt. Interestingly, this ancient recommendation is now validated by modern research. In addition to the above finding that exercise in the morning gives the greatest blood pressure drop during sleep, a recent study by Northwestern University sheds new light on the phenomenon of morning sunlight exposure and our health.

The researchers found that being outside in the morning appears to dramatically influence our metabolism for the entire day and those who get at least 20 minutes of outdoor light before noon weigh significantly less, even if consuming the same number of calories and controlling for sleep and other factors.

Researchers concluded that as much as 20 percent of our body weight is determined by how much morning light we get, which has a favorable effect on our metabolism. Our circadian rhythms get reset each day according to "sun time," when the first morning light is registered by brain cells in the supra-chias-mic nucleus of the hypothalamus. If we don't get enough light in the morning, our "head" clock in the hypothalamus, and the multitude of tiny "clock genes" in each of our body's cells that coordinate with it, become de-synchronized and our metabolism suffers.

One result may be, that even if we eat the same amount of food, we can tend to gain more weight. The researchers concluded that being outdoors in the morning at least 20 minutes is bene-ficial for weight maintenance. Add the extra benefit of walking outdoors to your morning "sun time," per the Ayurvedic sage Charak's suggestion, and you've got one doubly powerful tech-nique for good health!

Sitting Is the New Smoking: Uncomfortable News About Armchair Living

A sedentary lifestyle has become the American way. We live our lives sitting at computers, in class, in cars, at the movies, watching TV, attending meetings, playing videogames, texting, and surfing on our smartphones. We intuitively know that sitting so much isn't healthy, and now research demonstrates just how detrimental sitting can be to cognitive and physical health.

Cardiovascular risks aside, an important, oft-forgotten downside of sedentary behavior on both our physical health and cognition is loss of muscle mass. Since we women have less muscle tissue than men to begin with, we are at particular risk for "sarcopenia," a condition of atrophied muscles and reduced muscle strength. Maintaining optimal muscle mass via resistance training and proper nutrition helps prevent us from losing excess lean body mass and getting "frail"—an independent risk factor for dementia—as we get older.

And if you are more interested in losing weight than in avoiding frailty, lean muscle mass is important for you, too. The key point is that muscle tissue burns more calories than fat even when you're at rest. So the more muscle tissue you have, the more calories you'll burn, helping you maintain a healthy weight even with the same caloric intake and activity level.

Sitting and Your Brain

Researchers at the University of California, Los Angeles (UCLA) recently found that long stretches of sedentary behavior—like sitting all day at your desk—are linked to thinning of brain regions associated with memory, a frequent finding that precedes and coincides with cognitive decline, dementia, or Alzheimer's. Even before Alzheimer's disease steals memories, the condition starts to shrink the hippocampus and the entorhinal cortex, brain regions that lie at the heart of memory function.

More research is needed to see whether increasing exercise alone can restore volume in these key memory areas of the brain. Meanwhile, exercise is our best defense against brain shrinkage and cognitive decline, with at least 2 hours a week of regular exercise likely needed for significant cognitive improvement.

How Bad Are Weak Muscles for Your Brain?

One surprising cause of elevated dementia risk is "skinny fat," a condition of being normal or even underweight, but having weak, atrophied muscles and lacking in physical fitness. Fortunately, this brain-draining "skinny fat" condition can be reversed with exercise and strength training that rebuilds muscle mass, burns body fat, and results in a lower risk of brain deterioration.

Getting moving and building up your muscles has even more benefits, particularly for those already experiencing cognitive decline. Reducing sedentary behavior has been shown to improve cognition in those at increased risk for Alzheimer's.

Notably, Duvivier et al. found that just 4 days of slashing "sit time" back by 5 or 6 hours—substituting standing and self-reported light walking—improved cholesterol readings as well as markers of insulin sensitivity; i.e., lowered diabetes risk, including "diabetes of the brain".

Even if subjects continued to sit all day but added one hour of moderate to vigorous cycling-type exercise in the evening, cardiovascular markers such as endothelial function improved within days. It is encouraging, bordering on miraculous, to see that the body responds so quickly to our lifestyle—epigenetics in action—that even in the first few days of sitting less, your body already begins to get healthier!

If you have a desk job, I recommend that you do everything you can to counteract the effects of sitting for long periods of time. Get up and walk to the restroom, down the hall, or anywhere for 5 minutes every half hour or so. Unlikely to break so frequently? Opt for a standing desk and gradually work up to standing at least 4 or 5 hours of your day, plus walk around, even a bit, every time you can take a break.

I've used a standing desk myself for several years now and highly prefer it. You don't have to make a big investment to start, especially for work at home. For years, I used a couple of "banker's boxes" as an inexpensive computer stand that I could whip on top of my desk, or off it, anytime I wanted. There are also numerous excellent brands on the market if you have $150 to $300 to spend.

While I don't depart my desk frequently while I work, I add a few heel raises, knee bends, and push-ups against my desk when I feel a bit sluggish or am waiting for a page to load. It beats sitting and feeling impatient, and I feel fresher and more alert, not to mention stronger.

Don't strain to stand all day when you first get your standing desk. When you feel tired, sit. When sitting feels uncomfortable, stand up. You'll end up feeling more comfortable throughout the day. Studies indicate that standing at your desk increases productivity!

Most importantly, your health, mobility, and cognition in older age may depend on it.

Exercise Boosts Human Growth Hormone (HGH)

The HGH hormone is produced in the pituitary gland and is widely touted as an "anti-aging" hormone. Unfortunately, by the time we reach middle age our bodies are producing a fraction of what they produced when we were children. The reduction in HGH in the body is directly linked to poorer brain function. Celebrities commonly pay thousands of dollars each month for injections of growth hormone in hopes of maintaining their youthful appearance and physique. For those of us on a more limited budget, the good news is by exercising correctly, you can return your levels close to where you were in your 20s.

Exercise, including weightlifting and HIIT, boosts both HGH and a hormone called brain-derived neurotrophic factor (BDNF). BDNF is also like "miracle grow" for your brain and helps keep your mind and memory sharp. It is associated with increased intelligence, mood, productivity, and memory along with decreased risks of neurodegenerative diseases, including Alzheimer's and Parkinson's.

Weights Are for Women!

Lifting weights is a great way to keep your muscles strong, your bones strong, and to prevent the dangerous condition of frailty as you go forward into your later decades. As we've discussed, frailty itself is a major risk factor for cognitive decline, as well as low-bone density, poor balance, and weak muscles, increasing the chance of life-changing falls and fractures. The good news is you can keep yourself strong by systematically challenging your muscles and your bones with weightlifting.

If you wish to begin a weightlifting or resistance training program — and I highly recommend that you do — my main advice is to seek instruction in the proper way to do it. For example, when I first started working out years ago, I hired a personal trainer, sharing sessions with a friend to keep the cost down. I continued supervised sessions until I was confident, I had the correct form, knew my limits, and how to safely use any machines or devices.

You can sign up for two or three sessions with a personal trainer or health coach to get the hang of it. Tell your trainer that your top priority is to not get injured, as injury takes you out of the game and that is certainly a step backward. Get a trainer that truly understands that — possibly a woman will be more in tune with you and your body. If you don't have a trainer, read a book, go to YouTube, or ask a knowledgeable buddy to accompany you to your first gym sessions, and to help ensure you use proper form for each exercise.

In any case, you have to look out for yourself. Be mindful of your own body and your body structure. If you injure easily, take it extra easy, or get physical therapy to ensure you strengthen safely.

If you have trouble getting started, ask a friend or family member to help you, or better yet, train with you. Research shows we exercise more consistently if we have an "exercise buddy." Besides, you'll help your buddy improve his or her health, and what's not to love about that!

Manage Your Stress, Enjoy Your Life

The acknowledged founder of stress research, Dr. Hans Selye, defines stress as a set of physiological responses triggered by the perception of threat or challenge that mobilize the adaptive ability. The stress response is not bad as long as it turns on only when we really need it, and shuts off expeditiously, so cortisol is not produced in excess.

The body is designed to handle intermittent stress. However, when stress becomes chronic, excess cortisol can damage the memory centers of the brain, especially the hippocampus. Memory, long-term recall, and learning suffer. Chronic stress is a factor in most forms of cognitive decline and plays an important role in Type 3 (toxic) Alzheimer's disease.

Late nights, lack of sleep, skipping or delaying meals, worry, fear, anger, and excessive exercise all contribute to chronic stress. Alcohol consumption, tobacco usage, high fat, rich diet, lack of exercise, sleep deprivation, excessive caffeine (4 or more cups/ day) only add "insult to injury," exacerbating the negative impact of stress.

Studies show that the effects of prolonged or recurrent stress are damaging to the healthy functioning of the brain and body. In general, chronic cortisol secretion is at the root of the burnout and mental fog that many women and men experience at midlife. Add to that the effects of fluctuating hormones on the female brain during perimenopause and the need for truly effective stress relievers become self-evident. That is why stress reduction measures are critical to maintaining healthy brain cells and optimizing our cognition.

Natural Approaches To Managing Stress

Meditation, yoga, pranayama (a breathing technique), massage, biofeedback, prayer, contemplation, walks in nature, nurturing friendships, and music are all proven ways to calm the mind and reduce the damaging effects of stress on our brains, especially the hippocampal memory center.

When balanced and healthy, the hippocampus provides negative feedback to the adrenals and helps ratchet down stress hormone levels. When damaged by excess cortisol, the hippocampus loses this ability, exacerbating the vicious cycle of excess stress and cortisol excess. It's no wonder that stress can have a deleterious effect on mind and memory that only tends to get worse as we age—yet another reason to keep your stress in check with effective stress-management.

Meditation

Among the many ways to reduce stress, I have found Transcendental Meditation (TM) to be the all-around most effective for reducing stress in my patients. Even Ayurvedic routines, which can dramatically improve health, rarely produce the magnitude of response I routinely hear when patients learn TM and return to report their experience.

"It changed my life," with a big sigh of relief, is the most common phrase I hear. Indeed, transformations, including cessation of alcohol, drugs, and other addictions are common. Better sleep, relief from chronic headaches, PMS, arthritis pain and other health problems, less anxiety and smoother relationships with family and co-workers are also frequently reported. I've heard many times from grateful patients, that "things just don't 'get' to me the way they used to."

Among its many benefits, meditation reduces stress. TM and other forms of meditation have been documented to reduce excess cortisol, known to damage our hippocampus. There are many types of meditation: HeartMath, compassion meditation, mindfulness meditation, meditation apps, Transcendental Meditation, and others. I encourage you to find the one or more that appeal to you, and practice regularly, at least once a day. Consistent, regular practice "trains" the nervous system to adopt a new style of functioning, at a lower level of excitation and stress.

At one time, every meditation was considered equivalent. Like "meditation is good, just do meditation." This is akin to saying, "Pills lower blood pressure, just take a pill, any pill will do."

Comparison studies have shown that different meditation techniques yield different degrees and spectrum of benefits, depending on the type of meditation. To be more compassionate, compassion meditation may work best. To detach your mind from your emotions, mindfulness may work best. To achieve a deep state of restful alertness and relaxation, lower blood pressure, and calm the nervous system, Transcendental Meditation works best.

Dr. Travis and his colleagues were the first to identify three distinct categories of meditation; focused attention, open-monitoring, and automatic self-transcending and to correlate them with brain wave function. This created a much-needed mindshift regarding meditation in academic circles around the world. Just as no one pill cures all diseases, different meditation techniques result in their own unique range of benefits.

As a physician, I am in favor of whatever works for you. When a patient reports great benefits from their spiritual practice or meditation or relaxation technique, I am happy to know they have found and established a practice that benefits them, and I encourage them to keep it up.

The bulk of my experience over the past 40-plus years has been with Transcendental Meditation. I began my own personal practice of TM at age 16, and undertook professional training in meditation, becoming a certified teacher of Transcendental Meditation in Switzerland during a 9-month sabbatical following medical school at Johns Hopkins and before starting my residency at Stanford.

From an early age, I have been interested in the mind and its potential to promote health and healing. Becoming a certified teacher of Transcendental Meditation—the method that I had derived so much benefit from in college and medical school—was part of my professional plan to dive deeply into what meditation is and to integrate it into my practice for the benefit of my patients. Thousands of my patients have learned TM and I've had the pleasure of seeing how it nurtures them from within, dissolves their stress, and supports their healing journey in a multitude of ways.

Transcendental Meditation was the first meditation to be thoroughly studied scientifically, and that research provided me the confidence from a professional standpoint, to recommend it to my patients even 30-plus years ago.

Highly evidence-based, TM research preceded most other research on meditation by a decade or more, with the first studies appearing in Science, American Journal of Physiology, and Scientific American in 1970.

These now classic studies documented for the first time a "unique, hypometabolic state" of relaxed, alert mind, lower metabolic rate, slower heart rate, and decreased oxygen consumption. Researchers postulated this state to be a "fourth major state of consciousness" beyond waking, dreaming, and sleeping.

Since 1970, the National Institutes of Health in the United States has funded over $20 million of research studies on the Transcendental Meditation program, and hundreds of peer-reviewed studies have documented its benefits. Findings include lower blood pressure, less insulin resistance and metabolic syndrome, enhanced longevity, reduced anxiety, reversal of atherosclerosis, and a 48-percent reduction in mortality, heart attacks, and stroke in high-risk cardiac patients. Relevant to stress-reduction and brain health, studies have demonstrated lower cortisol, reduced PTSD and ADHD, and improved memory, learning, and brain wave coherence, a finding associated with a wide variety of psychosocial and behavioral benefits.

Most importantly, TM is easy to learn and to practice. It doesn't take a lot of time to "get good at it." It is common for people to have a deeply relaxing experience of inner peace, silence and deep rest right from the first meditation. Oprah, Dr. Oz, leading athletes and performers, and many other public figures have stated they practice Transcendental Meditation regularly, often after trying other forms of meditation without finding the inner peace from them that they were seeking.

More than one patient has told me, as this one, "I didn't think I could meditate. I tried so many ways. But TM really works for me. I just sink, like an elevator. I effortlessly drop into a deeply relaxed state."

For more information on TM, I recommend you read the excellent, New York Times bestselling book Transcendence, by NIH researcher and psychiatrist Normal Rosenthal, MD, or Strength in Stillness by Bob Roth for a terrific overview of the value of TM in your life.

You can also go to *www.tm.org* and read the research and watch the videos of the touching recovery stories of patients with PTSD, ADHD, anxiety, and more.

I have recommended TM in my practice to thousands of patients and continue to use it in my own life. As a result, I am confident that TM delivers the many benefits that nearly 50 years of research and hundreds of studies have documented. It is easy to learn and to practice.

There are scholarships and payment plans to make it accessible to nearly everyone. Celebrities, veterans, inner-city school children, world leaders, priests, rabbis, people of all faiths, Congolese refugees, world-class athletes, musicians, actors, and innovators practice TM. Why not you?

Breathing Techniques

Deep breathing exercises and alternate nostril breathing, aka "yogic breathing," both demonstrate a beneficial effect on the nervous system, calming down the "fight or flight" response and enhancing parasympathetic activity—our more relaxed, "rest and digest" mode.

Researcher Dr. Robert Freedman of Wayne State University studied the effect of daily deep breathing exercises in perimenopausal women and found that regular practice resulted in a significant reduction in hot flashes, probably through its effect on the autonomic nervous system.

You can multiply the benefits of deep breathing by applying the wisdom of yoga with a breathing technique called "pranayama." Pranayama is a Sanskrit term referring to any breathing technique from the traditional Vedic discipline of yoga intended to promote spiritual development and/or balance in the mind, body, or nervous system.

Research has documented that alternate nostril breathing reduces the stress response by activating the parasympathetic nervous system and inducing a relaxed state. According to Ayurvedic medicine, this simple technique also enables oxygen to penetrate deeply into the cells of the brain and the nervous system, energizing the brain and enhancing mental clarity.

How to practice alternate nostril breathing: First sit comfortably and place your thumb on your right nostril and close it. Breathe in through your left nostril. Then close off your left nostril with your third finger and release your thumb from your right nostril. Breathe out slowly and evenly through your right nostril. Next, breathe in through your right nostril. Now close your right nostril off and breathe out through your left nostril. It's traditional to change "at the top," after you have inhaled, before you change nostrils and exhale.

Here's how it goes: in, switch nostrils, out, in, switch nostrils, out ... breathe naturally and easily, not particularly deeply and not shallowly, not very slowly or very quickly. Take it easy and follow a comfortable rhythm. Repeat this cycle for about 5 to 10 minutes twice a day. Just before your meditation practice is a classical time of day to practice pranayama, as is right after doing a set of yoga poses.

I have a number of patients who attribute extended periods of pranayama twice a day—about 20 to 30 minutes each time—to significant improvements in their memory and cognition. One 80-year-old woman who recovered her memory after experiencing Alzheimer's symptoms following cardiac surgery thought pranayama would be boring but said, "I'm really grooving on it." Now, several months after fully recovering her cognitive abilities, she continues to practice pranayama 10 minutes twice a day for maintenance.

Brain Training: Use It Or Lose It

The search for the best mental calisthenics routine to stave off cognitive decline is a booming area of research and a multi-million-dollar business. Numerous scientific papers have shown the important cognitive benefits of brain training.

A recent study conducted by researchers at McGill University and Posit Science showed—for the first time ever in humans—that brain training can increase the ongoing production of a critical brain chemical that declines in Alzheimer's disease—acetylcholine.

Acetylcholine is a neuromodulator that the brain naturally produces when it needs to attend to information and is critical to memory and learning. Typically, the production of acetylcholine decreases with age, with more dramatic reductions seen in people with age-related cognitive decline, pre-dementia, and dementia.

The McGill pilot study involved a handful of older adults who did a brain exercise called "Freeze Frame" for about six weeks. At the end of that time, PET scans showed that subjects who had practiced "Freeze Frame" had increased levels of acetylcholine, as well as improved memory compared to controls.

It's the first time that brain training has been shown to increase acetylcholine in humans, and the news was received enthusiastically at the 2018 Alzheimer's Association International

Conference in Chicago. "These results are exciting and further validate many studies showing the benefits of targeted cognitive training to enhance attention," said Jerri Edwards, a researcher at the University of South Florida Medical School who has been studying brain training for more than a decade. "These results lend further credibility to our findings that specific types of cognitive training can reduce risk of dementia."

This is the second time in three years that brain training exercises have been highlighted at the Alzheimer's Association International Conference for their ground-breaking results in the battle against Alzheimer's. In 2016, results from a study that followed some 2,800 adults over a period of 10 years showed those who practiced a brain exercise called "Double Decision" had fewer car accidents, better executive functioning and as much as a 48 percent lower risk of dementia, depending on a variety of factors, including how long they had practiced "Double Decision." What is particularly remarkable, and motivating, is the finding that these benefits were still evident as long as 7 years later, even when subjects had not continued regular practice of the game!

Both "Double Decision" and "Freeze Frame" are commercially available to the public through a brain training website and mobile app called BrainHQ. I highly recommend that you check it out and commit to a regular schedule of playing these games. If you are losing memory or cognition, it is most effective to practice 10 to 20 minutes per day, five days a week or 30 minutes, three times a week. If you simply want to retain the good memory you have, I recommend you practice at least one day a week for 20 minutes just to "exercise" your brain cells in a way proven to prevent decline.

Many companies provide online brain training including Posit Science, Lumosity, Dakim and Cogstate. It helps to know that these training programs are set up to continue challenging you—as soon as you start doing well, they increase the difficulty.

Don't let it get stressful for you. Cut back on the time of each session, or try an alternative exercise for your brain, as I outline below. Brain training should be fun and fulfilling!

Brain-Training Recommendation:

Do brain training three times a week for about 15 minutes each time. Try *www.BrainHQ.com.*

Prefer To Stay off the Computer?
Check Out These Enjoyable Alternatives

Learning any new thing is also a proven way to keep your mind alert and counteract the effects of cognitive decline. You can learn a new language, learn to dance or play a musical instrument, start a new hobby, etc. In summary, to promote growth of your brain cells, cognitive skills, and memory, you need to reduce your stress level, challenge your brain regularly by learning new things and yet also give your brain some deep rest and rejuvenation.

Focus on your quality of sleep, stress management measures such as Transcendental Meditation, physical exercise, mental "calisthenics," proper organic, whole food and supplements, spices, and herbs to help nourish and flex your brain cells on a daily basis. In time, you'll find your senior moments transforming into flashes of deeper insight and creativity, inner wisdom, and greater enjoyment of life.

Take This Simple Action #6 Now!

Besides aging, stress is the most potent "hormone-zapper" we encounter. Yet, each of us reacts to stress differently and may benefit from some recommendations more than others.

Learn your unique "stress type," and how to minimize the effects of stress on your personal system by taking the short quiz at the link below:

www.thehealthybrainsolution.com/stress

You'll then receive one simple, personalized and highly doable "tip for your type" each week for six weeks. Integrate them one-by-one in an easy way to tame your cortisol, grow your resilience, and nurture your precious baby brain cells that are being born every day!

7

Detox your Brain—The Imperative

Epidemiologic trends suggest environmental
exposures (in) Alzheimer's disease.

—Suzanne de la Monte, MD, PhD

Key #7: Identify and Remove
Toxins and Their Source

The concept of "toxins" in the body used to sound like science fiction to my medically trained ears. However, my clinical experience of nearly thirty years has convinced me that toxic exposure and accumulation of toxins in the body lie at the root of many of today's health problems, especially seemingly unexplained symptoms. After all, our bodies are in constant exchange with the physical world around us. If that world is polluted, our bodies will also become polluted.

With the tremendous growth of industry over the past 100 years, thousands of toxic chemicals have been introduced into our food, air, drinking water, hygiene products, homes, cars, and just about everything that's manufactured. As a result, our bodies today are exposed to a potentially huge toxic load over a lifetime—a toxic build-up which can lead to type 3, or "toxic" Alzheimer's.

Type 3 is the most complicated and difficult cause of cognitive decline to treat. Deciphering the toxic causes in any one patient is akin to a private detective in a "whodunnit" movie, trying to uncover the perpetrators of a mysterious crime. Is it mold? Heavy metals, such as mercury from fish or dental fillings, arsenic from rice, cadmium from polluted soil? Or could it be a hidden infection such as Lyme, herpes, or Epstein-Barr? Is it air pollution, pesticides, herbicides, or other chemicals? The answer differs from one patient to another, and often there are multiple contributors, including genetically determined detox impairments.

When we find and correct one thing, we cannot rest easy. If symptoms do not clear, we have to look for yet another contributor. "No one loses memory for no reason," Dale Bredesen is fond of saying. It's an adage worth keeping in mind with type 3 cognitive decline, because those suffering from it are, far and away, the most challenging to turn around, and continued sleuthing over time is usually required.

Where Do They Come From?

Over 300 toxic substances have been documented in human blood samples, in umbilical blood, and even in breast milk, meaning our youngest and most vulnerable humans, with their sensitive, developing brains and immature detox systems, are being exposed. Equally concerning is the potential for damaging effects on future generations.

Recent research, in animals so far, indicates that the toxic effects of exposing a pregnant female rat to the popular weed-killer glyphosate a single time, extend as far as the second and third generation of her offspring. Researchers at Washington State University have documented a dramatic increase in prostate, kidney and ovarian diseases, obesity and birth abnormalities in these descendants, none of whom were directly exposed themselves. The bottom line is toxic chemicals have the potential to change our gene expression, and pass that on to future generations. Food for thought, indeed.

The here and now sequelae of many of these 300 substances include interfering with our hormonal systems and the nervous system, direct hits to our brain health. Some chemicals are non-degradable, such as PCBs, and accumulate in our bodies and brains over time, amplifying their effects and increasing the risk of neurodegenerative diseases such as Parkinson's and Alzheimer's.

Understanding that cognitive decline may be due to toxic exposure opens up new possibilities for successfully reversing it. In this chapter, you will discover to what degree toxins may have accumulated in your body over the years by looking at your symptoms. You will also learn how these toxins likely got into your body and ways to remove them in order to restore balance in your physiology. By "balance," we mean normal physiological functioning, the way the body was designed to function, with clear mind and vital body. And, as Ayurveda reminds us, balance is the key to perfect health.

Toxins and Your Brain

Research is continuing to accumulate that environmental toxicity is detrimental to the brain. A recent study carried out by Lilian Calderón-Garcidueñas, MA, MD, PhD, at the University of Montana found that growing up in a city with a high level of air pollution (Mexico City, in this case) can increase the risk of Alzheimer's disease. The study suggests that the disease begins much earlier than suspected in the context of such exposure. Elevated amyloid and tau levels, a precursor to Alzheimer's, were even found in babies less than a year old.

"Alzheimer's disease hallmarks start in childhood in polluted environments, and we must implement effective preventative measures early," said Calderón-Garcidueñas, a physician and toxicologist in UM's Department of Biomedical and Pharmaceutical Sciences. "It is useless to take reactive actions decades later."

The study concluded that exposure to high levels of the pollutant PM2.5 in air pollution was to blame. PM2.5 is a tiny particulate that is about 30 times finer than a hair follicle. These tiny pollutants come mainly from car exhaust and industrial, chemical, and power plants in cities where there is heavy smog, such as Mexico City, Los Angeles, Beijing and other similar urban areas around the world.

"Neuroprotection measures ought to start very early, including the prenatal period and childhood," Calderón-Garcidueñas said. "Defining pediatric environmental, nutritional, metabolic and genetic risk-factor interactions are key to preventing Alzheimer's disease."

Another study found that Alzheimer's risk in older women increased by 92 percent when they lived in cities where PM2.5 exceeded the U.S. Environmental Protection Agency's standard. Senior study author Prof. Caleb Finch, of the Leonard Davis School of Gerontology at the University of Southern California (USC), and colleagues say that if their findings apply to the general population, then PM2.5 could account for as much as a *full 20 percent* of dementia cases.

This is one cause of Alzheimer's that has definitely been "under the radar." I had never even heard of PM2.5 before researching for this book. Isn't it incredible that it may be causing one out of every five cases of Alzheimer's and we don't even know about it?

Characteristics and Symptoms of Type 3 Alzheimer's—"Toxic" Type

People with type 3 Alzheimer's, caused by chronic inflammation due to toxins or hidden infections, often have no family history of dementia and the most common genotype in this group, ApoE 3/3, confers no increased risk for the disease. Unlike other subtypes of Alzheimer's, type 3 does not begin with isolated, gradual memory loss. Rather, it usually starts more suddenly, following very stressful events such as divorce, loss of employment, or death of a loved one.

Symptoms of this subtype often include headache, depression, attention deficit, and difficulty accomplishing tasks such as problem-solving, organizing, planning, and even accomplishing simple mathematical exercises. The symptoms typically begin earlier than other types, in the late 40s or the 50s, around menopause (for women) and andropause (for men). Hormonal deficiencies aggravate this condition and restoring hormones to optimal levels is usually a necessary step in recovery from type 3.

What are the causes of this unusual type of Alzheimer's? What are the markers? And most important, are you at risk of developing type 3 Alzheimer's? A questionnaire on biotoxicity and a variety of blood tests can help you find that out. If your testing indicates you are at increased risk, there are steps you need to take to remove yourself from exposure and to detox your brain and body. Being proactive *now* can help prevent cognitive problems down the line.

Tests Help Identify Type of Exposure

Clues as to the cause of type 3 Alzheimer's come from extensive blood tests as well as MRI scans, which can reveal signs of "hidden inflammation" in your brain and body. (It's "hidden," because doctors don't usually check for it, and the usual hsCRP blood test that doctors *do* check doesn't usually reflect it.)

Pioneering doctor Ritchie Shoemaker, MD, first identified this type of insidious, low-grade inflammation as an indication of biotoxin exposure and environmentally acquired illness and coined the term "CIRS" (chronic inflammatory response syndrome) to describe its many symptoms.

CIRS-type inflammation can be caused by mold exposure, Lyme, viruses such as herpes, Epstein-Barr virus (EBV), heavy metals, and more. Most experts who treat type 3 Alzheimer's emphasize that type 3 is not *exactly* CIRS, but rather chronic, hidden inflammation that is causing cognitive decline. It's a bit of semantics. The most important thing to know is that type 3 is a subtype of Alzheimer's disease that inflicts its damage on the brain through a chronic inflammatory response to environmental toxins and infections.

Identifying the presence of this hidden type of chronic, "innate" inflammation is key. This is done by checking for markers of chronic activation of your innate immune system—the one that gets activated before specific antibody formation kicks into full gear to fight the infection or invader with more precise, targeted "bullets."

In some people, such as those genetically predisposed to poor antibody response to certain invaders such as mold, this first, non-specific immune response may persist, and become chronic, in a never-ending, ineffective attack on the enemy—a war that never ends. Chronic inflammation keeps the enemy partially at bay, but never completely obliterated, inflicting insidious damage year after year on the battlefield of your own bodily tissues.

It's critical to test for chronic, hidden inflammation and, if present, to identify and remove the cause—whether it be mold, Lyme disease, herpes virus, heavy metals, or another toxin. People don't get better, and the chronic, innate inflammation does not subside until the cause is removed. If you are found to have this type of inflammation, you will likely need the support of a doctor trained in the Shoemaker or Bredesen protocols, to sort out the cause and effectively treat it. Once corrected, the inflammation will gradually abate and corresponding markers in your blood will drop into the normal range over time.

What Tests Uncover Hidden Inflammation?

While there are a number of markers you can test for—each with its pros and cons—I usually recommend doing the TGF-beta1 as an initial screen, due to its relative affordability, sensitivity, and consistency across laboratories. Additional favorites of my colleagues in the field of environmentally acquired illness include MMP-9 and VEGF.

If the results of your TGF-beta1 test are above 2380 pg/mL, there is a good chance that you are being exposed to one or more aggravating toxins and your body is responding with chronic inflammation. In this case, I recommend you see a functional or integrative medical doctor who will guide you through a series of tests to identify the cause of the inflammation and help you eliminate the causes and recover your naturally healthy state.

Meanwhile, take the biotoxin questionnaire below and do a check on how you feel. If you are fatigued most of the time, are struggling with brain fog, have constant aches and pains, or don't have the energy you would like to feel, you may very well have hidden inflammation, infection, or toxicity.

Biotoxicity Questionnaire

Please circle any of the symptoms in the following list that you have been experiencing for more than the past two weeks.

General Symptoms:	• Fatigue • Weakness
Muscles:	• Aches • Cramps (especially claw-like cramping of the hands and feet) • Unusual pain (ice pick, lightning bolt, or electrical) • Joint pains • Morning stiffness

Unique Symptoms:	• Headache • Frequent urination and increased thirst • Night sweats • Static electricity or shocks • Appetite swings
Eye Symptoms:	• Light sensitivity • Red eyes • Blurred vision • Tearing
Respiratory Symptoms:	• Sinus congestion • Cough • Shortness of breath
Gastrointestinal Symptoms:	• Abdominal pain • Diarrhea
General Neurological Symptoms:	• Numbness • Tingling • Metallic taste • Vertigo • Temperature regulation problems • Dizziness • Tics • Atypical seizures • Fine motor skill problems
Central Nervous System Symptoms:	• Memory loss • Concentration difficulty • Confusion • Learning difficulties • Difficulty finding words • Disorientation • Mood swings • Anxiety or panic

Source: Richie Shoemaker, *Neurotoxicology and Teratology*, 2004.

How to Determine Your Score

If you have one or more symptoms in four or more of these eight categories, it is suggestive of chronic hidden inflammation such as mold or chronic viral infections, among others. The more symptoms you have checked, the higher the likelihood you are being or have been recently exposed to mold, other toxins, or infections.

MRI

An MRI is a brain scan that can detect shrinkage of the brain, inflammation of the neurons, and vascular leakage. An MRI sequence called FLAIR (fluid-attenuated inversion recovery) can help identify abnormal small white spots in different parts of the brain that are usually interpreted by the radiologist as "probable small vessel disease," but may also be seen in toxic exposures and type 3 Alzheimer's. Your doctor will order an MRI only if you have significant memory, cognitive, or other brain symptoms—it's not necessary to do for preventive purposes.

Are You Genetically Susceptible to Hidden Inflammation?

In addition to the ApoE4 gene type, there is another genetic predisposition to cognitive decline stemming from chronic inflammation, this time of the "CIRS-type" due to ineffective antibody immune response. This inherited susceptibility is bestowed by certain HLA (human leukocyte antigen) types, coded for by specific gene complexes. HLA genes make proteins that are present on most cells of our body and help our body distinguish "self" from "non-self." Depending on the type of proteins your body makes, your *adaptive, antibody-forming* immune response may work well (as is the case with an estimated 75 percent of us) or not so well (as with the other 25 percent) against certain invaders such as mycotoxins, bacteria, Epstein-Barr virus, and other infections. If your immune system's HLA type is in the less effective 25 percent, you may be more likely to react strongly to mold, develop chronic Lyme disease once infected, or suffer from chronic fatigue syndrome or other chronic, inflammation-promoting conditions.

You can find out your HLA genetic type through a simple blood test, though I don't routinely recommend it due to cost (from $350 to $750 depending on the lab) and the fact that it will not change the treatment and remedial measures you'll need to take if such inflammation is found. Nevertheless, if you're not well, it can be validating and empowering to you, and your loved ones, to identify any genetic vulnerability you may have. Armed with the understanding that you're not "crazy" or "weak" to have the symptoms you have can help bolster your resolve (and those around you), to do what it takes to ferret out the cause and undergo the often-involved process of healing from chronic inflammation and eradicating its underlying cause.

Beware of Ticks

One possible cause of hidden inflammation is Lyme disease. Many people are not aware that they have it. If you have a history of joint aches, rashes, and fatigue, be sure to get a Lyme screening test. Be aware that this is a controversial test, as many people who are found to have Lyme from more extensive testing, or simply are diagnosed with chronic Lyme based on clinical symptoms, may test negative on initial screening. Perhaps due to the fact that those who lack ability to form antibodies well to Lyme are the most likely to have it persist chronically, and yet these initial screens rely on finding the very antibodies they are not making.

If you live in a Lyme-infected area, take preventive precautions. Avoid walking in tall grass, fields, and other areas where you can easily get tick bites or acquire ticks. When you come in from outdoors, get in the habit of doing a careful and thorough tick check.

Remember also that the ticks most likely to carry Lyme are the very tiny nymph ones. They're hard to see and are most prevalent in the early spring when you might not be so alert for them.

Prevention is important and if you do notice a bug or bite on your skin that may look questionable, get medical attention right away. The signature rash of a Lyme tick bite looks like a solid red oval or a bull's-eye but may not be present in 20 percent or more with early Lyme. It can appear anywhere on your body. The bull's-eye has a central red spot, surrounded by a clear circle with a gradually expanding red circle on the outside.

If you catch a tick bite within the first 72 hours, just one dose of an antibiotic can usually wipe it out because it's still circulating in your blood, hasn't burrowed deep into the tissues and has not yet genetically changed to avoid the antibiotics that you're taking. You can often knock it out right away, so do see a doctor right away if you suspect you have been bitten.

I have a patient who contracted the disease by getting a tick bite just walking across her gravel driveway, albeit surrounded by tall grass, to get to her car. It is easy to contract where there a lot of ticks, especially in the springtime. Be sure to thoroughly check your clothing, legs, arms, scalp and neck, whenever you return home after a walk outdoors in Nature. Tossing your clothes in the dryer for 15 to 20 minutes upon returning home may kill any lingering ticks as well—not a bad habit to adopt if you are frequently hiking in Lyme-prone areas.

Are You Being Exposed to Mold?

Mold presents itself in damp, dark places, but also releases invisible spores into the air. You may not see them, but your lungs continue to breathe them. Are you being exposed to mold? Answering the following questions may help you become aware of an exposure you hadn't realized:

- Have you had flood in your basement? or water leaks in your house?
- Do you live in an old building with paint or old drywalls?
- Any corners of your house that have a musty smell?

- Do you have frequent headaches? Trouble with digestion?
- Do you suffer from allergies, chronic colds, or flu symptoms?
- Do people around you have chronic sinus problems?
- Do you live in a warm or cold, humid climate region?

Beware that 50 percent of the mold in your house is hidden—visual observations are just a starting point. Mold can hide behind drywall, in fabric, food, carpet, attics, and any other place susceptible to condensation. Mold often causes immunity problems and will present symptoms similar to a cold, flu or chronic allergies or sinusitis. The insidious black mold, *Stachybotrys chartarum*, can cause breathing difficulties, life-threatening pneumonia and bleeding in the lungs.

Mold toxicity has also been linked to neurological symptoms such as tremors, rashes, infertility, immunosuppression, and kidney toxicity. What many people don't realize is that mold can make you extremely sick, and even kill you. It can also be a major contributor to cognitive decline and Alzheimer's. Identifying whether you are being exposed, and whether your body is reacting to it, is of prime importance.

Testing for Mold—Do-It-Yourself Mold Kits

ERMI (Environmental Relative Moldiness Index)—The ERMI test is a DNA-based test that's used to identify specific species living in your home. By vacuuming (or using a Swiffer-type cloth) for an ERMI test, you can draw dust from one spot, or take from a variety of places around the home. The purpose of the ERMI cloth test is to identify and quantify any potentially pathogenic mold species present. This will help you know if you need to have any mold remediation done in your home. If mold exposure is the cause of your chronic inflammation and possibly your cognitive symptoms, removing it from your life is the first and most important step you need to take in recovering your health.

One of the simplest ways to order an ERMI test kit is from *www. momsaware.org*.

Testing for Heavy Metals

If you have evidence of hidden inflammation, you should also be tested for heavy metals.

High levels of heavy metals such as mercury, lead, cadmium, and arsenic are highly toxic, they can literally poison your brain cells while at the same time stimulating amyloid formation—your body's attempt to protect you. They block critical metabolic pathways including mitochondrial (your energy-producers) and those that help synthesize oxygen-carrying hemoglobin for your red blood cells.

Heavy metals poison the brain when they deposit in our nerve cells, damaging the mitochondria and slowing metabolism, one of the early dysfunctions that often precedes memory loss. Toxic metals can enter the body via consumption of food or water, inhalation of polluted air, or absorption through the pores of the skin. We can be exposed to heavy metals at work if we work in the agricultural, manufacturing, or pharmaceutical industries. We can also be exposed in older residential settings where lead paint was used.

It is important to know the most accurate means to test for heavy metals. A simple blood, stool, or urine sample will not usually show the presence of heavy metals unless you have been exposed to them within the past few days. Yet your body may have accumulated a big heavy metal load over time, shunting what isn't readily eliminated through the gut and kidneys into the body's issues, where they silently inflict their damage over time.

If you test high for heavy metals, I suggest you find an integrative or functional doctor who is familiar with chelation therapy. Chelation is a medical intervention to help eliminate mercury and other heavy metals from your system in a safe and effective way.

The doctor can prescribe a chelating agent, usually an oral agent will do. It will bind to the metals in your body, enabling your cells to extrude them so they can be carried out of the body through blood, stool, and urine. I often recommend the nutrient N-acetylcysteine, as it is gentle and well-tolerated, yet usually very effective. Coupled with dietary and Ayurvedic recommendations to support detoxification, chelation can be a relatively easy and comfortable process.

IV chelation is also available and effective. It may be preferable in some cases of extremely high levels but is usually expensive and unnecessary. Like oral chelation, it can strip out nutrient minerals at the same time as the heavy metals, so be sure your doctor is mindful to replenish them.

Mercury

Exposure to high levels of mercury can harm the brain, heart, kidneys, lungs, and immune system. As one of the volatile organic compounds (VOCs), mercury from old dental amalgams can become aerosolized and absorbed into the body. Long-term exposure to VOCs can cause damage to the organs and nervous system. A very sensitive test to evaluate the levels of mercury in your body is Mercury Tri-Test by Quicksilver Scientific. This test uses samples of hair, blood, and urine to assess for your body's mercury burden and its ability to eliminate it. If your level of mercury is toxic, it will identify the source, whether it is organic (from fish) or inorganic (from dental amalgams). You can order it online at *www.quicksilverscientific.com*. This company also offers tests for other heavy metals.

Lead

Memorably, in an article I once read on levels of lead in blood, the authors concluded, "No lead is good lead." Aptly put—no amount of lead is useful to the body, and any amount impairs cellular functioning and can diminish intelligence.

Yet lead accumulation is surprisingly common.

Getting the Lead Out: Memory Lost and Found

When I first saw Anne in consultation, she was concerned that she was "losing her mind." Her memory and mental clarity were steadily deteriorating, and she had trouble concentrating at work. An accountant for over 25 years, she worried she would soon have to give up her profession, even though at 56 years old, she had not yet saved enough to retire.

After ruling out depression, low thyroid, B12 deficiency, and several other possible causes of Ann's symptoms, I suggested testing for heavy metals. I explained that heavy metals can accumulate in the brain and nervous system and can interfere with mental clarity and memory, as well as causing other symptoms. It's good we tested, as her test results indicated a surprisingly high level of lead in her body. Lead, the heavy metal responsible for lowered intelligence in children, can also cause mind and memory problems in adults.

Since Ann's lead level was not in the very high range where intravenous medical treatment was necessary, I recommended a gentler and more holistic approach. First of all, I recommended Ann add spices, herbal detox support, and detox-supporting foods, including whey protein, to her diet. Next, supplements that support detox, especially of lead, were added, including a whole food-based multivitamin and mineral, vitamin C complex, a known lead chelator, and N-acetyl cysteine in a combination product shown to prevent re-entry of liberated heavy metals back into the brain. Ann also opted to undergo a series of the traditional Ayurvedic detoxification procedures MRT, followed by some Ayurvedic detox herbs along with her nutritional support, to help eliminate the accumulated lead from her body.

Three months later, Ann returned for a follow-up visit, smiling. Her mind and memory had "kicked in" again, and she felt she was back to her normal self. She was clear and focused, had no difficulty with her accounting and even took on new responsibilities at work. Repeat testing confirmed that her lead level had dropped into the normal range. Ann related that she planned to do MRT yearly to maintain her high level of energy and mental clarity, as well as continue Ayurvedic herbal support and occasional detox supplements for prevention.

Hair Mineral Analysis

Hair mineral analysis can show exposure to heavy metals over a period of several months, while a blood test typically shows more recent exposure. This test is considered by the U.S. Environmental Protection Agency as an effective test for the "biological monitoring of the highest priority toxic metals—lead, cadmium, mercury, and arsenic." The EPA also notes that "for toxic exposure ... [testing] hair appears to be superior to [testing] blood and urine." Note that if you dye your hair you should wait for at least two months to be tested to avoid contamination of the hair specimens. If your hair has elevated levels of heavy metals, you should see a doctor for further investigation and treatment.

Protect Your Mitochondria

Mitochondria are tiny cellular structures packed with enzymes and present in almost every cell in the body. They are our energy producers, our "power stations," as essential for healthy brain function as they are for whole body health. Mitochondrial enzymes take the foods we eat and the oxygen we breathe and convert them into energy. Since chemicals and toxins damage mitochondria, it is important to be aware of possible everyday exposures and take measures to avoid them as much as possible, especially if your genetics makes you particularly susceptible, such as those with ApoE4, or if you have impaired detox pathways. The list of potential and proven mitochondria-busters is long, including antibiotics, alcohol, Tylenol, heavy metals, pesticides, herbicides, household products, NSAIDs (aspirin, ibuprofen and related drugs), smoking, cocaine, methamphetamine, and others.

When your mitochondria aren't working properly, your metabolism runs less efficiently, and you may suffer from low energy and chronic fatigue. Neuropsychological changes are common, including "brain fog," mental fatigue, or spaciness in its milder forms, and if more advanced, confusion, disorientation, and memory loss.

The bottom line is that one of the ways toxins can damage your brain is by damaging your mitochondria. Take measures to avoid toxic exposures and fortify your body with nutrient-dense foods and supplements as needed, to support your body's natural protective and detox mechanisms.

Testing for Non-Metal Chemicals

Having practiced for nearly 20 years in Iowa, coined by a colleague "Monsantoville," due to its predominance of Monsanto-derived GMO corn and soy crops, I've noticed an ever-increasing frequency of crop dusting on land surrounding the small town of Fairfield where I've been living.

My observations are verified by official records tallying the annual use of pesticides and herbicides in Iowa.

I can't help but wonder if the steep rise in chronic diseases including cancer, Parkinson's, Alzheimer's, and other neurodegenerative diseases I'm seeing in my practice may be related to the local population's heavy exposure to agricultural chemicals.

The story of one of my patients, Genevieve, provides some initial supportive evidence.

Ever since moving to Iowa after retiring 5 years ago, Genevieve had suffered from a prominent facial rash that appeared every spring, lasted until November, and partially cleared in the winter, only to return full force again in the spring.

Genevieve lives across the street from actively cultivated farmland, where she reports observing planes dive-bombing the crops several times a month during "high" crop dusting season, from May through September.

Upon taking her pulse (Ayurvedically), I immediately saw a "connection" between the rash and an overload of toxins that her liver was struggling to process and eliminate. The skin, it turns out, has many of the same enzymes as the liver, and will "take over" detox functions when the liver is overwhelmed. My clinical impression was that Genevieve's liver was overtaxed by the annual chemical assault and her rash was a direct expression of her summer agricultural exposure.

Not satisfied with theory alone, I recommended Genevieve test herself for "non-metal chemicals," a simple urine screen.

Genevieve returned a month later with her report. True to her organic, vegetarian and clean "yoga" lifestyle, Genevieve tested low in all categories, except three—the three related to herbicides, pesticides and fungicides—the very chemicals being sprayed on the crops surrounding her house. In these three categories, she was over the 75th percentile, and in "organophosphates," comprised of 100 of the most common agricultural chemicals, she was "off the chart," above the 99th percentile. Ouch!

This test provided the objective confirmation Genevieve needed to remove herself in the summer, accepting her cousin's offer to spend summers in Vancouver with her. A pristine and beautiful place to enjoy the summer months! Genevieve also implemented a comprehensive detox protocol I prescribed, and now, two years later, her rash has finally disappeared.

Future testing has yet to be done, to verify that the chemical buildup is indeed diminishing. I fully expect it will, as Genevieve's skin is now clear and luminous, her eyes bright, and she no longer suffers from a variety of other minor complaints she had no idea were connected to toxins, including insomnia, anxiety, and lack of focus.

If you wonder if non-metal chemicals are disturbing your balance or robbing your mental capacities, I highly recommend you test for the level of non-metal chemicals in your body.

Remember, knowledge gives you the power to prevent harm and *optimize* your health, now and for the future.

Treatment

Treatment of heavy metal toxicity may take a few months if you have mild symptoms or several years if you're severely ill. Seek the guidance of an expert in the treatment of environmentally acquired illness using functional medicine, integrative medicine, Ayurveda, and other natural approaches if you have significant symptoms that don't clear with the recommendations in this book.

The first and most important step, and probably one of the hardest steps to do is to remove the source, even if it means *you* have to leave *it*, such as your mold-infested home, if only until it's remediated. The second step is to get those toxins out of your body.

Step 1: How to reduce or eliminate exposure to toxins in your environment:

- Water filter: Fluoride, chloride, and bromide are halogen gases commonly present in drinking water which can interfere with the usage of iodine by replacing it in the body. Get a water filtration and enhancement system that will remove unwanted chemicals and hardness and restore balanced mineral and pH levels to your water.

- Air filter: Select HEPA and activated carbon filtration system capable of capturing 99 percent of VOCs and 99 percent of all other pollutants.
- Fix your home: If there has been water damage, get any mold professionally removed by mold remediation experts. Mold can produce toxins that cause chronic inflammation. If lead is an issue, whether pipes or paint, seek professional advice about its removal.
- Avoid plastic: Plastic containers and plastic water bottles contain phthalates, among many other chemicals, which are endocrine-disrupting and toxic. Use glass instead.
- Use clean household products: Go to the Environmental Working Group's website (*www.ewg.org*) to find clean household products or buy your household cleaners from a natural food store or other "green" distributor.
- Buy toxin-free cosmetics: Most body care products and cosmetics are filled with chemicals, including lead. Did you know that 60 percent of any product you put on our skin is absorbed into the bloodstream? *Therefore, it is important to use toxin- free cosmetics.* Consult the Environmental Working Group's Skin-Deep Guide (*www.ewg. org/skindeep*). You will find a database of safe cosmetic products there to guide your transition to more healthful makeup and body care.
- Avoid artificial perfume, cologne, and sprays. These have been shown to poison not only the brain cells themselves, but their "efflux pumps," tiny structures that "pump" unwanted cellular substances, such as toxins, out of the cell. As in "get it out of here!" Unfortunately, perfumes containing "musk" chemicals (most of them) not only can

enter brain cells, but are *toxic* to the efflux pump, allowing the musk toxins to accumulate in the cells, and disallowing the cell's normal mechanisms from removing them. Avoid artificial perfumes (check out luscious tones of essential oil fragrances instead) and try to educate those around you of their hazards. You'll reduce your second-hand exposure and help them too!

• Detox your wardrobe: When clothes are treated with chemicals, such as in dry-cleaning, and then come in contact with our skin, some of those chemicals inevitably get absorbed. Hence, the importance of using non-toxic cleaning methods and of wearing natural fabrics such as 100 percent certified cotton fabric (preferably organic), linen, silk, wool, cashmere, or hemp.

Most synthetic fabrics are basically "plastic" fabric. In a process called polymerization, chemically derived fibers are joined together to create fabric. It requires numerous chemicals and solvents to create any type of synthetic fabric. Common synthetic fabrics include polyester, rayon, modal, spandex, and nylon. And just because your mother, grandmother, and her mother used them, it doesn't mean moth balls are safe. They are made of naphthalene, toxic to nerves, blood, and liver. They are classified by the EPA as Group C, a possible carcinogen—avoid them!

• Eat organic foods: Check out *www.nongmoshoppingguide. com* for a list of non-genetically modified and organic foods that are safe and good for your health.

To protect your environment and your own health from the effects of toxins, "reduce, recycle, reuse" should be your guiding principle. As for the toxins already accumulated in your body, the good news is that there *are* natural, scientifically tested ways to reduce your toxic load and accompanying health risks. Unlike chemical chelators, these natural programs do not run the risk of further toxic damage, *and* they are enjoyable!

Step 2: How to detox your body and brain:

There are two main ways that the body detoxes naturally:

Exercise: Exercise moves the lymphatic system which requires breathing and movement from the body's muscles to help move fluids and remove waste from the body.

Hand in hand with exercise is sweating, another major detoxification pathway of the body.

Hydration: Water is part of every metabolic process in your body. Adequate water intake ensures your kidneys have enough fluid to safely dilute and eliminate toxins from your blood. When feeling Thursday, always respond to your body's need. How much water should you drink? In general, you should try to drink between one-half to one ounce of water for each pound you weigh, every day. Ideally, drink at least ½ cup per hour. The best way to tell if your water intake is adequate is to check the color of your urine. A pure and healthy urine is light-colored and does not have a strong smell. If it's any darker then you need to drink more water.

There are also detox approaches that help the body eliminate excess toxins accumulated over time, which we will address shortly. But first let's look at Nature's self-cleaning program.

What is Detoxification?

Detoxification of chemicals is a fascinating story in itself. There are two biochemical steps or phases to neutralizing and transforming toxins to water soluble forms ready for excretion. Both phases are necessary in order to eliminate all types of toxins properly.

Phase I is carried out by enzymes called the "P450" system. Depending on the type of toxin, the P450 system of Phase I will either neutralize it and make it water soluble—at which point it gracefully exits the body—or make it even more reactive (and unfortunately more toxic) so that Phase II enzymes finish up the job of making it water-soluble and ready for excretion.

Phase II requires a variety of "conjugates," or "add-on" molecules that are attached to molecules made in Phase I, effectively neutralizing their over-reactivity and making them safe for the body to excrete without any collateral damage. Glutathione, sulfur, glucuronic acid, methyl groups, glycine, among others. Glutathione is an especially important detox enzyme we discussed in Chapter Two, that is made up of cysteine and two other amino acids, which are frequently in low supply in vegetarians and anyone who does not eat adequate protein or calories each day.

If Phase I is strong and Phase II is weak, you may be prone to even *more* severe reactions. This is because Phase I is preparing the toxins for Phase II by rapidly converting them into more highly reactive, more toxic substances and a weak Phase II can't rapidly eliminate them.

If both Phase I and II are slow or weak, then toxins generally tend to build up in your system and can cause chronic illness over time, including chronic fatigue, brain fog and many of the symptoms listed in the Biotoxin Questionnaire above.

To restate and simplify:

Some toxicants (the term for toxins from the environment) are easily flushed from the body as they are water soluble.

Other toxicants are fat soluble and easily get stuck in cell membranes or fatty tissues. They need processing before they can get out of the body.

For these stubborn, "sticky" toxicants, we have a two-step process of detox by the liver, aptly named "Phase I" and "Phase II."

Phase I enzymes make the toxicant more amenable to being flushed out; however, that means they can make the toxicant *more* toxic in the short run. (Side note: This step often produces free radicals—"bad guys"—that need to be neutralized too.)

Enter Phase II to save the day, by providing friendly small "conjugant" molecules like sulfur, methyl groups, glutathione, acetyl, and glucuronide that can then neutralize the toxicant and help it exit the body.

Important note: By the way, you only want to ramp up your Phase I activity if you have enough antioxidants on board, and a vigorous Phase II. Why is that crucial?

The logic is that we don't want to make our internal toxicants *more toxic* (as in "angry" or "irritable") by driving Phase I when we don't have enough soothing "juice" to neutralize and eliminate them from the body through a robust Phase II pathway.

Bottom line: Ingest foods that support *both* Phase I and Phase II pathways for best results. (See below for details.)

How Good Are You at Detox?

Your personal genetics partially determine how good you are at detoxing chemicals, including medications, drugs, caffeine, alcohol, and pesticides. People with certain SNPs (gene types) may have more limited ability to detox. Tests are available to test your detox ability, as well as your genetic endowment for detox enzymes. A functional medicine-trained doctor can help order those from a number of specialty labs for you.

It's very common, especially for vegetarians, to be low in nutrients essential for detox, and to suffer rashes, brain fog, fatigue, and other reactions to environmental exposures that their more nutrient-replete non-vegetarian friends handle without a symptom. My conjecture was verified by a highly experienced lab director, who noted the dozens of amino acid profiles I'd sent him from my vegetarian patients, nearly all with extremely low amino acid levels.

"Are your patients vegetarian?" he asked. "Yes," I responded. "And are they chemically sensitive?" Another "yes," from me. "I've seen this many times," he said. "Even in Asian countries, life-long vegetarians who are low in protein are chemically sensitive." Why is that? I suspect that chemically sensitive vegans and vegetarians aren't getting enough protein, including the key amino acid cysteine, to make adequate glutathione to protect ourselves from the onslaught of toxicants in our world today.

If you are vegetarian, be sure to boost your protein intake to at least 0.8 to 1 gram for every kg you weigh, (approximately 46-60 grams protein daily for a 135 lb. woman.) Also, take B vitamin and zinc supplements as well as a multi-mineral formula. Toxic buildup can happen to anyone, regardless of diet and lifestyle, yet I have found that ironically, those who are most "pure" and conscientious with their diet and lifestyle may unwittingly become increasingly susceptible to toxin damage, simply due to lack of nutrition.

Are You Chemically Sensitive?

Take a look at two common categories of chemical sensitivity, listed below as "caffeine intolerant" or "caffeine tolerant." If either apply to you, refer to the typical recommendations for each type listed below, which you can use as a guide. Regardless of your sensitivity level, by all means take precautions to fortify your detox system with adequate protein intake and nutrient-rich foods such as those listed below.

Self-Detox Approaches

For Caffeine Intolerant, Overly Sensitives
(You need to increase both Phase I and
Phase II detox, as below):

- Eat oranges and tangerines, caraway seeds and dill seeds (limonene containing, neutralizes carcinogens and enhances detox Phases I and II).
- Eat cabbage family vegetables daily (*brassica*). Cabbage, Brussels sprouts, broccoli, broccoli sprouts, bok choy, etc. (Increases Phases I and II).
- Take a B complex vitamin from whole food source daily (e.g., Mega food's "Balanced B").
- Get more high-quality protein in your diet if you don't already. Un-denatured whey protein is a good source of glutathione-building, Phase II-enhancing amino acids.
- Other Phase II enhancers are: Vitamin C, selenium, zinc, turmeric, fruits, vegetables, cooked fish, asparagus (rich source of glutathione). Ideally, get these in whole foods, or in whole food supplements if needed. Oral glutathione is not absorbed and is not recommended, unless in the more expensive, "liposomal" form.

For Caffeine Tolerant, Overly Sensitives
(You need to increase Phase II, but not Phase I, as listed below.)

- Turmeric—use a pinch of this spice in everything you cook (capsules of turmeric, or its "active ingredient," curcumin, may be fine, but be aware that they may over-stimulate the liver and gallbladder, according to Ayurveda). Turmeric is an amazingly useful and powerful spice that both enhances Phase II and tones down overactive Phase

I reactions. In addition, it has strong antioxidant, anti-in-flammatory and anti-cancer effects.

- Quercetin (found in many fruits), clove, and grapefruit all reduce Phase I hyperactivity. If reactions are very severe, try drinking 1 cup grapefruit juice daily in addition to your other recommendations. This reduces Phase I reactions by 30 percent. (Check with your doctor before doing this if you are taking hormones, contraceptives or drugs prescribed by your doctor, since grapefruit intake can change your blood levels by affecting liver detox of the medication.)
- Take a B complex vitamin from a whole food source daily (e.g., Mega food's "Balanced B Complex")
- Get more high-quality protein in your diet if you need it. Un-denatured whey protein (organic or from New Zealand, which is organic-equivalent,) is a good source of glutathione-building, Phase II-enhancing amino acids.
- Other Phase II enhancers are: Vitamin C, selenium, zinc, turmeric, fruits, vegetables, cooked fish, asparagus (a rich source of glutathione). Ideally, get these from whole foods, or whole food supplements, if needed. Oral glutathione is not absorbed and is not recommended, unless in the more expensive, "liposomal" form.

  Note: If you have a medical condition, check with your doctor before taking any food supplement. This product is not intended for the diagnosis, treatment or prevention of disease and has not been approved by the FDA. Keep in mind that as your body eliminates more toxins from the tissues, your kidneys, liver, and bowel have to deal with them. The Detox Tips below are designed to support and protect your elimination organs as they process and excrete the toxins that were liberated.

225

Detox Tips

The Western and Ayurvedic general detox tips below are designed to help keep your body metabolizing and eliminating well. A six-week detox is ideal, but even a week or two can help.

- Drink ½ cup of boiled warm-hot spring water every hour until 6 p.m. to help open the circulatory channels and flush out toxins. You can also drink the detox tea as well (see recipe below).
- Add fresh ginger root to your daily diet. A thin slice with a dash of rock salt and lemon before the meal will stoke your detox fire.
- Strictly avoid any cold or iced drinks, ice cream, frozen yogurt, or other cold foods and drinks. Favor warm, cooked, freshly prepared foods that are light and easily digestible, such as a more vegetarian diet of soups, vegetables, and lightly cooked grains like couscous, quinoa, and barley.
- Cook at home as much as possible.
- Use a pinch of turmeric—a superstar purifier for the liver—in your cooking along with fennel, coriander, cumin, and fenugreek. (See the Smart Spice detox recipe below.)
- Fresh probiotic sources such as homemade lassi or kefir.
- Fresh steamed or sautéed greens like chard, kale, dandelion, and mustard. Greens stimulate bile flow.
- Cabbage-family vegetables including kale, broccoli, cauliflower, and broccoli sprouts.
- Tangerines and other citrus fruits containing limonene.
- Fish oil (highly pure only).
- Onions, leeks, and garlic (sulfur-containing foods).
- Avoid cheese, yogurt (except as lassi, a fresh yogurt drink), cold foods and drinks, including ice cream and other frozen desserts, red meat, chocolate, sugar, and alcohol.

- Regularly take steam baths, saunas, or infrared saunas to induce sweating, an important avenue of toxin elimination. Ayurveda recommends placing cool, damp cloths over the heart, head, and the forehead during heat treatments, to prevent the brain and heart from overheating, a source of imbalance and stress for those vital organs, in particular.
- Exercise regularly to the point of sweating, if not medically contraindicated. Average at least 2 hours per week to significantly benefit your brain.
- Try to get more rest, especially by going to bed early to take advantage of the body's natural cleansing cycle from 10 p.m. to 2 a.m.

Your Smart Spice Detox Recipe

Use ½ to 1 teaspoon daily with lunch and dinner for 6 weeks. Note: All measurements in the box below are teaspoons.

Smart Spice Detox Mix
Fennel 6
Cumin 4
Coriander 4
Turmeric 2

Instructions:

Measure the number of teaspoons listed for each of the ingredients above. If it does not add up to at least 14 teaspoons, double each amount. Ideally, use whole seed when available, and grind fresh in a spice/coffee grinder every two weeks. Store all powdered spices in an airtight container and keep in a cool place away from direct sunlight.

To get the full benefit of both water-soluble and fat-soluble fractions of these spices, do both of the following at lunch and dinner each day. This combined approach brings out the optimum healing properties of the spices.

To get full benefit from the water-soluble fraction:

Mix ½ teaspoon of your personal spice mix with soup or cook in with your grain or vegetables. If you do not prepare any grain in water or vegetables, at least sprinkle lightly toasted spices over your food at the table (see "for meals away from home" below).

To get full benefit from the fat-soluble fraction:

Add ½ teaspoon of your spice mixture to one tablespoon of melted ghee (clarified butter) or pure, organic, cold-pressed virgin vegetable oil, and heat over low to moderate heat until aroma is apparent. Drizzle spiced ghee/oil over your grain or other dishes just before serving. (Avoid overheating the oil, indicated by "smoking," to prevent degrading the oil and forming unhealthy fat byproducts.

For meals away from home:

Stir the spices in an ungreased pan over medium heat until lightly browned. Then put in a small container and carry with you. Sprinkle on your vegetables or other dishes when you eat out during the day.

Detox Wise Water™ Recipe

This custom herbal "tea without the tea leaves," enhances the detox process. For example, coriander seeds are mildly diuretic and improve urinary flow. They also have action directly on the liver, helping to induce glutathione production and other biochemical pathways important for detoxification. Fennel and cumin gently support the digestive and post-digestive processes, helping prevent gas formation and stress to the gut and liver from poorly digested food.

Detox Wise Water
¼ tsp coriander seeds
¼ tsp fennel seeds
¼ cumin seeds

Boil 1½ quarts (6 cups) of pure spring water or safely filtered water for 5 minutes. Pour into a thermos. Then add the following spices in whole seed form to the thermos of freshly boiled water. Be sure to use organic spices.

Drink the water throughout the day. If you like, allow the water to cool to warm or room temperature after pouring into glass, before drinking. Simply drink the water and do not eat the ingredients themselves. The water-soluble fraction of the spices will be helpful, but the other parts may be aggravating for your system.

You may drink plain, room-temperature water during the day according to your thirst but try to drink all your Detox Wise Water by 6 p.m. Drinking it later may interfere with sleep due to its diuretic effect.

This Wise Water must be made fresh every day, and the thermos thoroughly washed and scrubbed with hot soapy water after each use.

Further Options For Biochemical Support:

I have found the following supplements helpful in protecting the body during ongoing exposure and aiding in the elimination of accumulated toxins.

Note: As always, if you have a health condition, please check with your personal health care practitioner before beginning any supplements, and before making major diet or lifestyle changes.

- Coconut charcoal—in capsules. Binds toxins in the gut and prevents them from being reabsorbed, which can easily happen if you have an overgrowth of "bad bacteria."

Coconut charcoal is usually well tolerated but may mildly loosen the stool. You can take two capsules at bedtime or 2 to 3 hours before or after meals or supplements. (Note: charcoal tends to bind any compounds in the gut to prevent their absorption, so better to avoid taking it around the time of food or other supplements.)

- Bentonite clay—in capsules. "GI Detox" by Bio Botanicals is a favorite brand of many environmentally literate doctors. It contains both clay and charcoal, whose loosening effect tends to balance out the mildly binding effect clay has on the stool. The purpose of clay, as with charcoal, is to bind toxins in the gut and prevent "bad bacteria" from acting on them in a way that promotes their reabsorption. Taking additional fiber daily as well as a good probiotic is helpful in this regard as well. If you wake up in the night feeling vaguely but decidedly uncomfortable during a detox program, likely you need to boost your gut support with either of these two products, in addition to checking out your microbiome, the balance of gut bacteria to see if you have an overgrowth of "bad bacteria," yeast or parasites. One of my patients cured both her insomnia and her sugar cravings when her occult parasitic infection was finally diagnosed and treated successfully. (She took an antibiotic specific for parasites; however, botanical products are also successful in some cases.)

- Liposomal glutathione is a supplement that provides a bioavailable source of the body's most powerful, endogenous antioxidant, combating the effects of physical and emotional stress, pathogens, toxins, free-radicals, and aging. Start slowly, with no more than one capsule per day, and work up as tolerated. Releasing too many toxins at once can lead to symptoms.

- N-acetylcysteine has an antioxidant and anti-inflammatory effect in the body. It supports liver detoxification and provides cysteine, an important building block of glutathione. Whey protein also supports detoxification through similar mechanisms. Be sure your whey protein is organic and you keep the amount in balance. Usually 20 to 25 grams per day is adequate and doesn't overload the digestive system or liver.

Ayurveda Herbal Support for Detox

The three main herbals for this self-care detox are traditional Ayurvedic combination formulas that help prepare the elimination system of the body for smooth and comfortable detox. I've chosen these three because they are premier Ayurvedic detox formulas and my experience has shown they are generally well-tolerated by the vast majority of individuals, if used in the manner described below.

Herbal #1: Genitrac

"Guduchi" or "heart-leaved moonseed," *tinospora cordifolia* is the star detox ingredient of this formula, as it is described in Ayurveda as promoting the removal of both internally generated and environmentally acquired toxins. The Genitrac formula also contains amalaki, a multi-purpose rejuvenative that notably supports digestion without aggravating pitta (the heat dosha). Note: guduchi is also present in "Elim-Tox O," found on *mapi. com*, along with complementary herbs, such as *manjistha* (*rubia cordifolia*) that "cools" the liver and skin and provides additional diuretic action to help flush toxins out through the urinary tract.

Usual dose: One to two tablets of this herbal formula may be taken daily. Or add it to the detox tea recipe above, where it will dissolve into the water and deliver a steady, but gentle detox support throughout the day. If you experience too much diuresis

231

(you feel you're urinating more than is comfortable during the day), cut back the dose to one-half to one tablet per day.

Herbal #2: Digest Tone

This formula is classically known as "Triphala," a combination of three fruits that are revered in Ayurveda as rejuvenative for the eyes and skin, as well as promoting long life and reversal of aging. The formula has a gentle, mildly laxative effect, supports elimination of excess cholesterol and fat-soluble toxins through the bile, and has dozens of other benefits according to the Ayurvedic texts. Recent research found that Triphala has an anti-mutagenic effect and may lower the risk of pancreatic cancer.

Mapi's Digest Tone also contains a rare, very potent, and effective form of haritaki that makes Digest Tone especially effective as compared to other versions of commercially available triphala. Lastly, Mapi adds the herbal cabbage rose for an extra soothing effect on the mind and emotions, as well as reducing excess "heat" sometimes associated with purification.

Usual dose: One to three tablets at bedtime is the traditional dose and time of administration. It is especially helpful if elimination is slow or enhanced cleansing is desired.

Herbal #3: Amrit Kalash—Nectar Tablet

This formula, as you may recall from Chapter Two, is the most powerful rejuvenative formula described in the Ayurvedic texts, and dozens of published research studies have verified its health-promoting effects. One of the most powerful, well-balanced antioxidant formulations ever tested, Amrit helps protect the body from the damaging effects of free radicals generated on a daily basis in the body's cells and tissues. In addition, Amrit is particularly valuable after a detox program has been completed, to strengthen and renew the tissues, making them more resistant to aging, free radical damage and toxic accumulation in the future.

Usual dose: One tablet twice a day. Available at *www.mapi.com.*

A Traditional Whole-Body Ayurvedic Rejuvenation Program

Long ago, Ayurvedic medicine predicted that accumulated toxins could be removed through specific detoxification procedures. Over 5,000 years later, modern scientists decided to put this prediction to a test. Using high tech laboratory studies, Robert Herron, PhD, and John Fagan, PhD, conducted a two-month longitudinal study on 15 subjects using Ayurvedic detoxification procedures, including 5 days of a standardized form of *panchakarma treatment,* called "MRT™" treatment, along with a special purification program before and after the treatment.

Treatment consisted of ingesting ghee daily for several days prior, which helps soften and dislodge fat-soluble toxins, mild laxative therapy to enhance gut elimination, and then 5 days of whole body oil massage, whole-body heat treatment such as a steam "bath," or warm oil poured all over the body, and finally, a daily enema, alternating water-based with oil-based, again to promote elimination through the bowel.

The results in terms of reduction of toxic load were highly significant. Compared to before treatment, blood levels of the highly toxic substances PCBs and beta-HCH were reduced by 46 percent and 58 percent respectively. Without this detoxification program, the expected drop in PCB and beta-HCH over a two-month period is only a fraction of one percent.

No previous method has been scientifically verified to reduce levels of these fat-soluble toxins in the human body without causing negative side effects. Normally, these fat-soluble substances remain in the body for many years. It is quite striking that nearly

50 percent or more can be removed from the blood in just 5 days of treatment.

To put the findings in a broader context, it is worth noting that there are two categories of toxins found in the human body: water-soluble and fat-soluble, i.e., stored in water versus fatty tissues, respectively. Most of the chemicals that have been linked with cancer and other serious disorders are *fat soluble* toxins, such as PCBs, PBDEs and numerous pesticides. Non-Ayurvedic detoxification approaches such as steam baths, saunas, aerobic exercise, and other activities can reduce water-soluble toxins substantially through perspiration and drinking large amounts of water.

Unfortunately, these strategies do little to remove the fat-soluble toxins that are sequestered in adipose tissues throughout the body and have been associated with a wide range of health problems from reproductive disorders and diabetes to several types of cancer, and more recently, Alzheimer's disease.

The MRT program on the other hand, has demonstrated the removal of *both* types of toxins and appears to be especially effective in removing fat-soluble ones that are otherwise very difficult to eliminate.

The MRT program uses a variety of non-toxic, lipophilic (fat-dissolving) materials, such as clarified butter in the purification diet, as well as herbalized sesame oil applied externally through massage and oil bath treatments. The Ayurvedic texts describe that these traditional methods sequentially loosen and remove lipid-soluble toxicants from their deposited sites and stimulate their excretion.

Ayurveda Nourishing Self-Detox

Fundamental to self-care in Ayurveda is the regular practice of self-massage with herbalized oil, called abhyanga. It is a gentle, nourishing procedure that you can do yourself at home.

When done in the morning, when your body naturally is eliminating, abhyanga (rhymes with "I'll be younger!") provides a kind of natural, home version of "MRT" detox. Ayurveda describes that massaging your whole body with oil nourishes your skin, moves the lymph and helps dissolve and mobilize toxins that accumulate in the body and skin over time. Sesame oil has potent anti-inflammatory effects and has been shown to be neuroprotective in animal models of Parkinson's disease, preventing brain inflammation and loss of neurons in response to toxin exposure. It also improves circulation, relaxes the mind and the body, and nourishes all the tissues and organs. Specific oils (olive, coconut, almond, and sesame) are selected according to your skin type and which *dosha* you wish to balance.

Note: The use of organic oils is preferable since they do not introduce dangerous chemical residues or trans-fatty acids into your body.

Which oil should *you* use?

Sesame is described in Ayurveda as the most purifying and healing, and the best overall for massage. Use sesame oil if you tend to run "cold," have cold hands or feet or just don't have any particular sensitivity. However, if you are prone to skin irritation, you should use coconut oil as it is the most soothing, cooling, and non-reactive. Olive oil is a good option with many of the same benefits as sesame oil, for example, helps prevent skin cancer, and is anti-inflammatory. Opt for olive if you do not like sesame for some reason, and coconut feels too cooling for you.

Oil Self-Massage Instructions

The best time for your oil self-massage is in the morning before taking a bath or shower. This helps promote the natural elimination pattern of the body in the morning. Alternatively, do your abhyanga in the late afternoon or early evening, before your evening meal, to help dissolve tension.

Warm up your oil by selecting a small squeeze bottle or a small container of it, in hot water, in the sink. When the oil is warm, you are ready to begin. Sit on an old towel in the middle of your bathroom. Use the flat of your hands for the entire massage, which is essentially an application and rubbing in of the oil. Apply a small amount of oil to the body, starting with the scalp all the way down to your toes.

Start massaging your scalp slowly with firm pressure. After two minutes, move down to your ears and face using small circles. (If you are prone to breakout, skip the face, or use coconut oil, which is least likely to irritate.)

Then start with the left shoulder in a circular motion. After a few circles, follow with long strokes on the upper arm, circles on the elbow and long strokes on the forearm. Do a few circles around the wrist and then long strokes up and down on the hand. Repeat with the other arm.

Use circular strokes around your breast and abdomen and upward strokes on your lower back.

Continue on to the left leg, by doing circles on the hips, long strokes on the thighs, circles on the knees, up and down on the lower legs, circles on the ankle, long strokes on tops and bottoms of the feet, and lastly, use your thumbs to massage up and down and in-between your toes - bliss! Repeat with the other leg.

Your feet should get special attention. Foot massage is a very important part of abhyanga. Ayurveda holds that it not only benefits the feet but revitalizes the whole body. It increases energy, balances emotions, and improves blood and lymph circulation. By massaging the nerve endings in your feet, you help release stress and relieve aches and pains.

Your Nose—The Gateway to Your Brain

According to Ayurveda, the nose is the gateway to the brain. The downside of this is how easily air pollutants can enter the nasal circulation, travel straight into the brain and accumulate, stimulating amyloid-beta production and leading to "inhalation Alzheimer's," a newly recognized cause of cognitive decline. However, the *upside* has been known and used for thousands of years by Ayurveda, including sniffing herbalized oils in the nostrils one or more times each day.

The ancient textbook of Ayurveda, the *Charaka Samhita,* claims that "one who does oil sniffing regularly, does not age in the head, and the sense are well-maintained." Not age in the head, not lose sight or hearing? Validating research yet or not, *I'm in!* How about you?

I suggest you give it a try and see how you feel. The use of oil in the nose (*nasya*) lubricates the nasal cavity and helps maintain moist sinuses, supports immunity and potentially protects from pollen and environmental pollutants. Some of my patients have reported the practice alleviates and prevents headaches, eases sinus pressure, and makes them less reactive to airborne irritants. Ayurveda describes that regular application of oil in the nose relieves dryness, calms and nourishes the nervous system, eases tension in the head, neck, throat, and jaw, and fosters calm, stable energy.

Ideally, use sesame oil, the best all-around healing oil according to Ayurveda. One of my favorite herbalized sesame oils for the brain is "Nose-to-Brain Oil" by the Anti-aging Company, available online. It contains nourishing herbs for the brain including *shankapushpi*, an herb held in Ayurveda as the best overall support for mind and brain function.

Directions:

Wash your hands thoroughly

Put 1 to 2 drops of oil on the tip of your pinkie finger.

Insert your finger into your nostril and rub the oil into the nose.

Pinch your nostrils and while closed, start to sniff in, creating negative pressure, i.e. potential suction.

Release your fingers as you continue to sniff up. The oil will be pulled further into your nostril.

Repeat with the other nostril.

Do once in the morning and repeat later in the day if desired.

Note: Avoid nasya when pregnant, just after a meal, just before bed, feeling ill, or if experiencing an acute sinus infection.

Final Note on Detox

Detox is a vast topic and functional medicine experts have effective protocols to promote it, involving many supplements and often advising the use of infrared saunas. This is a valid approach to detox and has helped countless individuals regain their health.

I have found great benefits combining the traditional Ayurvedic detox approaches with judicious use of supplements and diet to ensure that the body is nutritionally equipped to effectively detox. If you have toxic symptoms that do not resolve with the recommendations in this book, I certainly would advise you to seek out the input of a professional with knowledge of integrative or functional medicine, and ideally Ayurveda as well.

Now, turn to the next chapter for a summary of all seven keys and what steps to take for each, to set you on your path to staying sharp, on or off hormones!

I hope to see you on my online courses (see *www.myagelessbrain.com*), in my Healthy Brain Consultation Program, in my office, or on one of my upcoming My Ageless Brain retreats. Check out the many ways we can interact at *www.drnancyhealth.com*.

Until then, I wish you the best of health, an ever-sharp mind, a happy heart and a long, fulfilling life!

Take This Simple Action #7 Now!

Ready for a quick health and beauty transformation with the most fundamental, evidence-based health practices from Ayurveda?

Radiate health and vitality quickly with my complimentary online "Seven Days to Radiant Health and Ageless Beauty" program here:

www.thehealthybrainsolution.com/transformation

Your Seven Keys to Staying Sharp

50 years old is the time to do your colonoscopy,
40 years old is the time to do your "cognoscopy."

—Dale Bredesen, MD

Your Easy-to-Follow, 7-Step Program

In my practice, I have found that Ayurveda and the Bredesen Protocol work hand in hand to identify and treat the causes and mechanisms of Alzheimer's disease. My observation aligns with that of Bredesen and his colleagues—it often takes 4-6 months of "living the protocol" to stop or reverse cognitive decline, though I have seen patients get better in as little as two weeks or take as long as 9 to 12 months to get better.

Depending on your time and budget, I recommend you implement these seven steps gradually over time. Adopt a pace that works for you to fully implement each "key" before you move on to the next. I suggest the sequence below, but feel free to pick whichever key you feel drawn to start with.

A good strategy is to pick the item you think will be easiest for you to do. However, I strongly encourage you to get as many of your "cognoscopy" labs as possible from the start, because the results will empower you with self-knowledge as you address each of the seven keys presented in this book.

Once you know your "vulnerable points"—such as low hormones, B12 deficiency, high mercury levels, or inflammation—the relevant key takes on greater significance to you. Did you find out your sugar handling is poor? You may feel highly motivated to change your diet and even give up your afternoon cookie binge. You would also want to get the gluco-keto-meter to watch your blood sugar improve as you adopt a lower carb diet, Mediterranean diet, up your exercise, and reduce your stress.

Once you have integrated the first key as part of your daily routine of life, it will be easy to add the next one. Take seven days, seven weeks, or seven months to integrate these seven keys, in the way that works best for you. I've described it as a seven-month program. But if you already notice cognitive changes, it's prudent to integrate all seven keys as quickly as possible, without stressing too much, since time is of the essence to prevent further loss.

Also, if you are retired or have time in your schedule, implement them as expeditiously as your routine allows, again, without pressuring yourself. Some keys will get integrated more quickly than others. Approach it easily and begin to enjoy the overall health benefits you are sure to notice as your actions create the foundation for a healthy brain and good memory for many years to come.

Month One

Key #1: Identify and Remedy Your Risks

Find out your areas of vulnerability

1. Get started on your "cognoscopy," the full battery of tests to identify your vulnerable areas and to guide you and your doctor in correcting and optimizing them. Go to *www.thehealthybrainsolution.com* for a free, downloadable, printable PDF that lists the Comprehensive Lab Tests that I typically recommend to my Healthy Brain Program patients. You'll want to bring a copy to your doctor or use it to guide your ordering of test kits online. You'll also

find a scaled-down version, called the "Basic Lab Test List" which itemizes those tests I consider the minimum essential starting point, usually available through your doctor. These lists also contain *optimal* lab values for each test as cited by leading experts, the levels recommended for optimal brain benefit, not simply the accepted "norm" for the population provided by the lab.

2. Find out your ApoE type. The result will let you know if you are genetically at increased risk of late-onset Alzheimer's disease. This test is no longer such a scary proposition. It used to be that people would say "why do I want to know? There's nothing I can do about it, and I'll only worry!" On the contrary, knowing that you have one or more copies of ApoE4 today, along with the preventive knowledge in this book, can help you stay motivated to do what you need to do to stay mentally sharp and brain-healthy. What's outlined in the coming chapters will help you stay cognitively and physically vital for a lifetime.

   ApoE4 has another powerful "silver lining." Carriers of 1 or 2 copies of ApoE4, the increased susceptibility gene, tend to respond fastest to this protocol. In other words, this protocol usually works well for ApoE4 carriers, and even more quickly than for non-carriers.

   Remember, your genes are *not* your destiny. Take appropriate measures now to protect your brain health and your "epigenetics" (the genes you activate with your healthy lifestyle) can win out.

   Fortunately, Medicare usually covers this test for purely screening purposes, so you might get coverage with no other diagnosis than simple screening. You can also order the ApoE genetic test online, for self-pay, at:

   □ *www.MyApoEscore.com.* $199; includes specific subtype of each allele.

- *www.23andMe.com.* $199 or less. Simple "yes/no" to ApoE4. Upside is that it includes additional genetic information that you can upload to other sites to learn about your genetic detox capacity (i.e., *www.geneticgenie.com*) and other interesting facts about your genome.
- *www.lifeextension.com.* $198; includes specific subtype of each allele. Lab tests through this site are often deeply discounted in April and May during their "Annual Lab Test Sale."
- *Note:* It's preferable for your doctor to avoid using the diagnosis "memory changes," or "mild cognitive impairment," etc., if you may wish to apply for long-term care insurance. (Even "insomnia" can be a disqualifying "red flag" to them, according to some sources.) These diagnoses can permanently disqualify you, given today's insurance climate.
- Also, you may prefer to acquire long-term care insurance before testing your ApoE status. An Alzheimer's research subject recently informed me that all subjects in her study were advised that insurers are not restricted on what questions they can require on applications and that ApoE4 status may be a disqualifier. (This is very unfortunate, since knowing your ApoE status can be helpful in *preventing* you from ever getting the disease, through changes you are motivated to make in your lifestyle, etc.) It is your decision, of course, and I want to be sure you have all the information possible to make the best one for you. Genetic counseling may also be available to you through major university medical centers, to aid you in your decision.

3. Establish a habit of doing brain games three times per week for 15 minutes or so. If you prefer, do shorter sessions five days a week. The main thing is to enjoy it and

play it as any game. I recommend BrainHQ due to the large volume of research that documents its lasting benefits for memory and brain health. However, what's more important than which site is to play them regularly. Any site you enjoy and will do regularly is fine! See *www. BrainHQ.com.*

If you don't enjoy online activities, choose another way to learn something new and challenge your brain. Learn a new language, pick up dancing as a new hobby, learn to play the guitar or an instrument of your choice. There is evidence that each of these activities helps protect memory and cognition over time.

4. Assess your memory. If you want to know how your memory measures up, or you have any concerns about your memory, or *others* have told you *they* do. I suggest you take the Montreal Cognitive Assessment (MoCA). It is a simple, straightforward, verbal, paper-and-pencil test that assesses several cognitive domains: attention and concentration, executive functions, memory, language, visuo-constructional skills, conceptual thinking, calculations, and orientation.

5. You'll need a partner you feel comfortable with to administer it to you, as it involves remembering and repeating back words, simple calculations and other tasks. It is freely available online for download and takes about 15 minutes to do. (Available at *http://dementia.ie/images/ MoCA-Test-English_7_1.pdf.*) A normal MoCA score is 26 to 30; a score of 19 to 25 is associated with MCI (mild cognitive impairment). Scores lower than 19 suggest dementia. See your doctor if you score less than 26 or feel you would have aced it a few years ago and now you found it more difficult than you expected (subjective cognitive impairment).

6. Be sure to bring your test order sheets with you to your doctor to be sure you get as comprehensive an evaluation

as possible, right from the start. (Download free at *www. thehealthybrainsolution.com.*)

7. Dr. Bredesen has an online program called the "ReCODE Report," which will take your test data and analyze it using a computer algorithm. It generates a report that includes an assessment of the vulnerabilities you have in terms of a percentage value for each of the Alzheimer's subtypes: Inflammatory, Glycotoxic, Atrophic, and Toxic. It also provides you with a personalized diet, supplement, and behavioral program based on your results. There is a fee involved and not all recommended tests are included, but it is a good starting point if you are unable to pursue testing and treatment with a Certified Bredesen ReCODE Practitioner. See *https://www.ahnphealth.com/recode.html* for details.

Summary of Tests for Your "Cognoscopy"

You can get convenient order forms to take to your doctor or to guide your online test kit ordering at *www.thehealthybrainsolution.com*. Each form includes a brief description of the purpose of each test and optimal values for each.

You'll get access to two forms, one "Basic," that itemizes the most important tests to do to get started, even on a limited budget, and one "Comprehensive" list if you can do all of them from the start.

Table 1 is a simplified listing of tests for your Cognoscopy:

Table 1	
Category	**Tests**
Genetics	ApoE

Table 1	
Category	Tests
Inflammation	hs-CRP Homocysteine Omega-6:Omega-3 ratio A/G ratio (albumin:globulin ratio is part of "CMP below; no need to order separately) Body mass index (BMI; use online calculator) Oxidized LDL Cholesterol, HDL, Triglycerides, LDL particle number, small dense LDL Glutathione, total Gluten sensitivity (serum gliadin ab) Optional: celiac panel; autoantibodies panel; cross-reactivity gluten, grain panel (Cyrex lab); serum zonulin (leaky gut)
Insulin Sensitivity and Glucose Control	Fasting insulin, fasting glucose, Hemoglobin A1C (HgA1C)
Nutrients and Hormones (Trophic support)	Vitamins B6, B12, and folate Vitamins C, D, E RBC thiamine pyrophosphate Vitamin D Estradiol (E2), progesterone (P) Pregnenolone, DHEA-sulfate Cortisol, morning (by 9 a.m., ideally) Total testosterone, free testosterone TSH, free T3, free T4, reverse T3 Ferritin (iron stores, which can affect your memory and productivity if low, as many women are, especially if vegetarian)

Table 1	
Category	**Tests**
General	CBC (complete blood count) CMP (complete metabolic panel) Urinalysis with reflex culture and sensitivity (many postmenopausal women have urinary infections they are unaware of, this can affect cognition especially in the elderly. I order a urinalysis for all women presenting with cognitive symptoms.)
Toxin-related	Mercury, lead, arsenic, cadmium (Ideally, do these with a doctor who will give you a chelating agent beforehand to increase chance of finding heavy metals stored deep in your tissues.) Copper:zinc ratio TGF- B1 Optional: VEGF, MMP-9, MSH, HLA-DR/DQ
Minerals (if not included as toxins)	RBC-magnesium (red blood cell, not serum) Copper, zinc Selenium Potassium Calcium
Cognitive performance	CNS Vital Signs (via your doctor) MoCA (in doctor's office or with companion) Informal self-assessment with online games such as BrainHQ or equivalent
Imaging	MRI with volumetrics (only if you have noticeable decline)
Sleep	Sleep study (can do a home sleep apnea test available online—you'll get use of a device that measures your oxygen level during the night)

Table 1	
Category	Tests
Microbiomes	Gut, oral, nasal (gut, if you have digestive complaints or have taken multiple antibiotics; oral, if you have less than ideal gums or dentition; nasal, if you score high on TGF-beta1 or other markers of chronic innate inflammation)

Month Two

Key #2: Balance Your Inflammatory Response

Check your parameters:

- Do you have inflammation in your blood? Test your high-sensitivity C-reactive protein (hs-CRP) level to see if you have inflammation that can be damaging your arteries. If elevated, you will need to take steps to eliminate the inflammation—relax, it's mainly a wholesome diet! (See Chapter Two.) Since inflammation is one of the most important drivers of cognitive decline, you'll want to put out the "fire" as quickly as possible. Diet is key.

- Are your arteries narrowed? Are you at risk of heart attack? The MESA calculator gives you a "best estimate" of your risk of heart attack in the next 10 years. It is available online and is free. (For greatest accuracy, get your "coronary artery calcium score" done with an "ultrafast CT scan" of the heart and coronary arteries. This test is often available at very low cost for self-pay at a hospital in your area. Ask your doctor for a prescription for this test if you have increased risk of heart attack; i.e., have elevated blood pressure, cholesterol, diabetes, or pre-diabetes.)

- Check your blood pressure—take the average of three readings over one week. If the average is 130/80 or higher, see your doctor for evaluation, and remember, keeping it below 120/80 has added value for your cognition down the line.
- Test your omega 3 and 6 levels. Your ratio should ideally fall between 0.5 and 3.0. Omega-6 promotes inflammation. Omega-3 is anti-inflammatory and is directly nourishing to brain and nerves. Omega-3s, especially DHA, support mood, memory, and overall brain and body health. If you have ApoE4, supplement with krill oil, fish roe, or by eating fish two to three times per week for best absorption.

Reduce your inflammation:

- Manage stress: The body's acute response to stress can help us rise to challenges and perform at our peak, but too much destroys the hippocampus, a key memory center. How are you handling stress? Do you have a particular stress style? Find out with a short and simple quiz: Go to *www.drnancyhealth.com* and scroll down to the stress quiz banner. Take the short quiz to find out your "stress type" and you'll get one tip for your type each week to help soothe your nerves and ease your stress. It's Ayurvedically informed and refreshingly beyond "the usual."
- Favor an anti-inflammatory diet, low in refined carbohydrates, high in soluble fiber, high in mono-unsaturated fatty acids, a higher omega-3 to omega-6 ratio, and high in polyphenols found in colorful fruits and vegetables. Include Mediterranean diet staples such as organic olive oil, wild-caught fish, and abundant fruits, vegetables, walnuts, flax, and legumes. (See Chapter Two for details.)
- Avoid deep-fried foods, refined carbs, processed foods, non-organic and GMO foods, non-essential over-the-

counter medications, excessive alcohol, recreational chemicals, and smoking.

- Learn meditation to calm your mind. Find a practice that works for you. For example, consider adding meditation such as Transcendental Meditation to your daily routine. TM is a scientifically validated meditation technique that's doable and relaxing even to those who say they "can't calm their mind or sit still."
- Exercise daily. Start an exercise routine and stick to it. Get a buddy, hire a trainer, join a class, or find something you really love—like learn to dance, take your dog on longer walks, or whatever will keep you active.

Month Three

Key #3: Heal Your Gut and Better Your Brain

Stoke your digestive power:

- Your gut health is a powerful determinant of your immune system balance—whether you are inflamed or not. Use well-known dietary factors and Ayurvedic wisdom to help heal your gut and improve your digestion.
- Take the Digestion Type Quiz to find out your dominant "dosha" digestive type. Go to *www.drnancyhealth.com*. Scroll down the home page to the digestive quiz banner. The quiz is just a few questions long. Based on your answers, you will be learning your current digestive type and will receive an individualized tip for your type once a week for six weeks. This is a great way to integrate personalized gut tips from Ayurveda that's fun and doable.
- Start to incorporate the personalized healthy gut recommendations you will receive each week based on your quiz results.

- Diet: Eat fresh, organic, whole, non-genetically engineered (non-GMO) foods. Cook at home as much as possible to control the quality and freshness of what you are eating. Ideally, buy and eat only organic foods, rather than taking in more toxins like synthetic pesticides and herbicides with every bite. If you can't afford *all* organic, avoid the "Dirty Dozen," and favor the "Clean Fifteen." You'll readily find lists of these online.
- If you have digestive symptoms that don't clear up with these tips, see your doctor for a checkup. If they find nothing wrong, you may wish to consult with a functional medicine doctor or take a few steps yourself. First, you can begin to take probiotics and prebiotics.
- Reminder: Probiotics are beneficial bacteria that are good for your health. Prebiotics are non-digestible food ingredients that promote the growth of beneficial microorganisms in the intestines. If that's not enough, you may want to check your microbiome to see if you have imbalanced flora, yeast, or parasites—see Key #5, below.

Optional steps to optimize digestion:

- Take some probiotics and prebiotics. I suggest starting with a "sporebiotic" for optimal absorption and colonization of the good bacteria you're taking in.
- Test your microbiome. Find out if you have enough good bacteria or too many of any unwanted bacteria or yeast in your gut. You can get a test without a doctor's order online or ask your functional medicine doctor for a more complete test that includes parasites and markers of digestive function. *BiohmHealth.com* is one online service that will map your good and bad bacteria and give you an idea of your microbiome status.
- Eat the largest and heaviest meal of the day at noon, when your digestive power is at its strongest. This will prevent

the buildup of *ama*, or toxins. Do not overeat. Ayurveda recommends leaving one-third of the stomach empty to allow digestion to do its work. It's thoroughly mixing the food with enzymes, acids, and secretions. That doesn't happen smoothly when we've stuffed it full! Avoid cold water (especially with ice) before, during, and after a meal, since it reduces the efficiency of digestion. If you're thirsty, sip small amounts of warm water with the meal. Warm water with a squeeze of lemon is both delicious and stimulating for your digestion.

- Cultivate the habit of remaining seated for about five minutes after you've finished eating and before getting up and resuming your activities. This gives digestion a good start.
- Here's one of the most powerful, yet simple, techniques I've found in all my years of practice. Gifted to me by a revered Ayurvedic mentor, who received it from his grandfather physician-mentor, it is the simple act of drinking boiled, hot spring or purified water throughout the day for several months. Aim to drink about 4 cups of boiled warm to hot water daily, taking at least a few sips every half hour, to promote hydration, improve digestion and elimination, reduce cravings, balance menstruation if still happening, and promote elimination of impurities from your body.

Month Four

Key #4: Optimize Your Blood Sugar

- High insulin and high glucose are two of the most important risk factors for Alzheimer's. Be sure to test your fasting insulin and fasting glucose levels, as well as your HgA1C, a measure of your average blood glucose over the past two to three months.

    ☐ Results for the fasting insulin level should be 4.5 µIU/ mL or below and fasting glucose level should be 90 mg/dL or lower.

- Your HgA1C should be less than 5.6 percent.
- Extend your food-free interval in each 24-hour daily cycle. Adopt what is called the "Ketoflex 12/3" lifestyle. Establish a minimum period of 12 hours of no calories between the end of dinner and the beginning of breakfast and 3 hours of no calories before going to bed. This "intermittent fasting" helps shift your body into ketosis (burning fat for fuel), which has been shown to lower the risk of developing Alzheimer's and helps the brain heal from cognitive decline that has already set in.

  Note: Around 10 p.m., if not already in bed, you may start to feel hungry. However, know it to be a "false hunger," a sign of your metabolism revving up to digest the leftover wastes and food byproducts from the day. Your body isn't asking for food, assuming you had at least a light meal earlier in the evening. On the contrary, your body is designed to houseclean after 10 p.m., clearing out metabolic wastes and toxins, including cleaning the lymph channels of the brain and performing autophagy — eating up wastes and impurities accumulated in the cells. Resist the temptation to eat. Drinking a glass of boiled hot water at this time can relieve the hunger and will help your body do its "housekeeping" tasks more effectively.

- Diet: Avoid refined carbohydrates and foods with added sugars or corn syrup, including "organic and natural" sugars, because they still raise blood glucose levels. Eat at least a half a plate full of organic, non-starchy vegetables at lunch and dinner, plus nuts, seeds, legumes, whole fruits, adequate proteins, and healthy fats. (See guidelines for the Mediterranean style eating in Chapter Two.) Add turmeric, ginger, cinnamon, and fenugreek to your meals. Drink "Be Trim" tea by VPK Herbs or take *Gymnema sylvestre*, two capsules with each meal, to reduce sugar absorption and help reduce cravings.

- Turn your light off by 10 p.m. and strive for 8 hours of uninterrupted sleep. When you are asleep by 10 p.m., the brain and the body make optimal use of sleep for rejuvenation. Give it a try and see how fresh, radiant, happy, and energetic you feel when compared to a late bedtime. (See tips for good sleep in Chapter Six.)

Month Five

Key #5: Correct Your Nutritional Deficiencies

- Keep your brain healthy by nourishing your body and brain, providing it with all the growth-supporting nutrients it needs to flourish, and getting oxygen-rich blood pumping through it with regular, invigorating exercise.
- Test your vitamin levels of B12, B6, B9 (methylfolate), and vitamin D, as well as vitamins C, E, and RBC-thiamine. Check your minerals as well: serum copper, zinc and selenium, and RBC magnesium (must be "RBC," not serum). Calcium and potassium will be checked as part of your comprehensive metabolic panel, an inexpensive survey of your kidney and liver function, among others. Optimal levels of these vitamins and minerals are important for optimal brain function.
- Eat the right amount of protein in your diet. The general rule is "listen to your body," and use non-vegetarian foods as a "condiment," not the main course. Think "Chinese stir fry" for approximate proportion of vegetables to flesh

foods. (See Chapter Five for details.) If you are vegan or vegetarian, ensure that you are getting *enough* protein—deficiency *can* be an issue, even if you are not aware of it.

• Take brain-boosting supplements based on your test results. If your homocysteine is high, then vitamin B12, methylfolate (which is more bioavailable than folic acid), and B6 (pyridoxal-5-phosphate) are in order. Ask your doctor to advise you if you have a medical condition or take medications. Consider supplements to support your mitochondria, such as alpha-lipoic acid, PQQ, nicotinamide riboside, resveratrol and ubiquinol, and citicoline to support your acetylcholine levels (if not on Aricept or similar medication). Check out Ayurvedic brain health superstars: bacopa, gotu kola and ashwagandha which help curb amyloid production and nourish and help rejuvenate your nerves. (Visit *www.mapi.com* for a reliable source of Ayurvedic supplements.) Use turmeric daily in your cooking and consider curcumin capsules, especially if your inflammation level is high.

Month Six

Key #6: Restore Optimal Hormone Levels

Are your hormones in balance? Test your levels of estradiol, progesterone, DHEA-sulfate, and pregnenolone using serum blood tests. Remember, if you are taking hormones topically (through the skin), test the relevant hormones using a saliva or blood spot (capillary/fingertip stick) for most accurate results.

Consult your doctor or functional medicine practitioner to prescribe appropriate doses and make sure you have periodic serum, blood spot, or saliva results if you choose to take hormone therapy or supplements. Direct your doctor to the website of ZRT Lab (*https://www.zrtlab.com/sample-types/saliva/*) to learn more about evidence-based optimal testing methods for each route of hormone delivery.

- Test your thyroid hormone: testing should include the following: TSH, free T3, and free T4, and if you can afford the full panel, include reverse T3 as well.
- For women: if your partner is taking testosterone, regularly check your own testosterone level since cross contamination is common. Excess testosterone may disturb your overall hormone balance, as well as create unwanted side-effects such as facial hair growth, irritability, and thinning of hair on the head.
- Exercise boosts the hormone called brain-derived neurotrophic factor (BDNF). This hormone keeps your brain young and sharp. Introduce short bursts of maximum output exercise during your training sessions. For example, alternating 45 seconds of easy pace with 15 seconds of "all out." Aerobic exercise with bursts, such high-intensity interval-training, may create added brain and metabolic benefits over same-pace sessions. Aim for the minimum amount of exercise shown to protect cognition—2 hours total each week.
- Get 8 hours of good quality of sleep. Keep a consistent sleep schedule by going to bed by 10 p.m., even on weekends or during vacations. Get up at the same time every day (by 6 a.m.), for maximum energy, alertness and productivity during the day. (See more tips in Chapter Six.)
- Establish and maintain daily measures to manage stress. If you haven't adopted a specific stress-reducing approach yet, consider attending an introductory session at your local TM center, yoga studio or try an online app for relaxation.

- If you haven't started already, add brain exercises 3 times a week for 15 minutes. Play *Double Decision* or *Freeze Frame* on *BrainHQ.com*.
- Learn something new this month! If you're a workaholic and learning new things constantly, invest time in learning how to relax. Spend time with your kids or grandchildren, do something fun or romantic with the love of your life, or take an all-day outing to hike and picnic in nature.

Month Seven

Key #7: Identify and Remove Toxins and Their Source

- Toxins are the cause of type 3 Alzheimer's. Find out whether your body is harboring heavy metals, chronic viral infections or Lyme disease, fighting mold or is otherwise taxed by toxins. Removing toxins helps restore optimal mitochondrial function, critical to correcting the hypometabolism and mitochondrial dysfunction that lies at the core of Alzheimer's-related metabolic processes.
- Assess your likelihood of toxicity by taking the Biotoxin Questionnaire.
- Test your TGF-beta 1 to find out if you have hidden inflammation or infection. If the result of your TGF-beta 1 is above 2380 pg/mL, your body may be dealing with hidden toxins or infectious agents. See a functional doctor to identify and correct the cause of this type of inflammation.
- Check yourself for clues to chronic innate inflammation or undiagnosed infections. Are you fatigued most of the time? Struggling with brain fog? Do you have constant aches or pains? Do you have enough energy throughout the day? If so, see your doctor for a checkup. If he or she declares you "healthy" and your symptoms continue, see

an integrative or functional medicine-trained physician for further evaluation.

- Test your environment for mold. If you have high inflammation, a high score on the Biotoxin Questionnaire, chronic sinus or nasal congestion, or asthma or shortness of breath, order a mold testing kit online and be sure to check your TGF-beta1. I recommend the ERMI home mold test kit available at *www.momsasware.org*.
- Consider getting tested for heavy metals and be sure to do so if you feel you have any memory or nervous system issues. Get the help of a trained practitioner to guide you through a "challenge test" using a gentle chelator to pull heavy metals out of your tissues so they show up when you test for them. You'll also need a practitioner to help you remove them from your body safely and fully.
- Take steps to remove toxins from your environment: for example, get water and air filters, professionally remove any mold, buy green, non-toxic household products, and so on. (See Chapter Seven for more tips.)
- Start using the Ayurveda home nourishing detox program: oil massage and nose lubrification. (See Chapter Seven.)

Remember! It can take up to a year of following a comprehensive, customized program, including these seven keys, to stop or reverse cognitive decline. The steps listed in this chapter are a summary of select changes you can make that may have a *big* impact on your risk of Alzheimer's and will help you optimize your health and memory starting today.

Conclusion

This book was born to provide you with evidence-based, healthy brain solutions to stay sharp and healthy in a most natural way. I hope you now understand the underlying causes of Alzheimer's and how to identify and correct your personal vulnerabilities.

You now have a "road map" of the seven key areas of brain health and how to optimize them to safeguard your mind and memory for a lifetime. Integrating these seven keys in your daily life will not only reduce your risk of cognitive decline but will sharpen your mind while boosting your overall health.

You have also gained the ability to discover your digestive and stress "types" and receive personalized tips to balance your gut, calm your nerves, energize and optimize your metabolism, eliminate your exposure to toxins, cut your stress and sleep better—all based on the latest evidence-based research and time-tested Ayurveda.

My sincere wish for you, and every woman over 40, is to live a long, healthy life, overflowing with vitality in mind and body. May every passing day expand your heart and mind and your ability to love, fulfill your purpose and contribute all the good you can to this fragile, yet beautiful life on earth.

Take This Simple Action Now!

Go to *www.thehealthybrainsolution.com* and download your free, printable PDF of the Comprehensive Lab Tests I typically order for Healthy Brain preventive evaluation.

You can bring a copy to your doctor or use it as a guide to ordering self-test kits online. This one easy step will set you on the path of healthy, sharp mind and memory for a lifetime.

www.thehealthybrainsolution.com

Would You Like a Healthy Brain Consultation with Dr. Lonsdorf?

Contact us at 641-469-3174 or *healthoffice@drlonsdorf.com*

Resources

Services with Dr. Nancy Lonsdorf

For a private consultation with Dr. Lonsdorf, please contact us at 1-641-469-3174 or *healthoffice@drlonsdorf.com*. Dr. Lonsdorf works intensively with a limited number of patients seeking optimal brain health, guiding your progress with a highly personalized program informed by the Bredesen protocol, functional medicine and her 30+ years of experience integrating Western medicine with Ayurveda.

My Ageless Brain™ 12-Episode Webinar Intensive

Learn online with Dr. Nancy, access in-depth expert interviews, and implement your own "healthy brain" program with Dr. Lonsdorf's self-study video course: *My Ageless Brain; 7 Keys to Staying Sharp*, at *www.myagelessbrain.com*. For a time-limited $100 discount to readers of this book, enter "HBS108" at checkout. Dr. Nancy will guide you through the 7 keys in a 12-episode course, plus bonus interviews with experts in hormones and the brain, heart health, mold, and other environmentally acquired illnesses, meditation for optimal brain function, and *more*. Includes a special bonus interview with Kristin, Dr. Bredesen's "Patient Zero," the first person ever documented to recover from Alzheimer's.

Take the Quiz!

Find out your "stress type" and "gut type." Go to *www.drnancyhealth.com* and scroll down and click on the quiz banner of your choice. You'll get a "tip for your type" each week for 6 weeks to help you integrate healthy diet and lifestyle actions according to your own mind-body needs.

Download Your Lab Test "To-do" List

Get organized for your "cognoscopy." Get your Comprehensive, or Basic, Lab Test "to-do list" at *www.thehealthybrainsolution.com.*

Ayurveda Personal Wellness Online Course

Learn how to care for your mind-body balance on a daily basis, directly from Nancy Lonsdorf, MD, and Stuart Rothenberg, MD, including how to take your own pulse for self-healing, with this lively "take at your own pace," online course.

A full panel of self-quizzes are included to help guide your progress. In addition, you may opt for a series of sessions with your own personal Ayurveda wellness coach, to help you implement your Ayurvedic wellness program and enjoy the greatest benefits. See *www.ayurveda-courses.org.*

Integrative Ayurveda Health Professional Training

Are you a health professional, yoga teacher, or coach? Learn Ayurveda from physicians with more than 60 years of combined experience in this delightful, profound, and eye-opening training. You'll quickly be ready to apply the basics to benefit your clients, patients, self, and family. This course is self-study, at your own pace. Certification in Maharishi Ayurveda Level One training is available once you complete the course and all assessment tools. See *www.ayurveda-courses.org.*

This course also comprises the introductory level training course of a distance education master's degree program at Maharishi University of Management, online. For more information, go to *www.mum.edu.*

The Raj Ayurveda Health Spa

The Raj is an in-residence spa that offers complete, authentic Maharishi Rejuvenation Treatment (MRT) under the supervision of an Ayurvedic expert with a doctorate in Vedic Medicine. Offers scientifically documented detox and rejuvenation programs for a wide variety of chronic health disorders, as well as for overall stress reduction, anti-aging, beauty, and spiritual development.

1734 Jasmine Avenue
Vedic City, IA 52556
1-800-248-9050
www.TheRaj.com

The Transcendental Meditation Program

Contact the nearest center teaching the Transcendental Meditation program in the United States or Canada at 1-888-532-7686 (1-888-Learn TM) or email *info@tm.org*. Check out the latest research, as well as inspiring videos of meditation benefiting the lives of those with PTSD, ADHD, and anxiety, as well as enhancing the lives of high performing individuals. *www.tm.org*.

Maharishi Ayurveda Products, and VPK Herbals (USA)

For information on obtaining Ayurvedic wildcrafted and organic herbs, spices, and other products mentioned in this book, call Maharishi Ayurveda Products International (MAPI) at 1-(800) 255-8332 or visit *www.mapi.com*.

Maharishi Ayurveda Products and Ayurvedic Herbals (UK and EU)

www.maharishi.co.uk
+44 (0) 1695 51015
info@maharishi.co.uk

BrainHQ

BrainHQ is an online cognitive training system designed by an international team of neuroscientists. The exercises both assess and improve attention, processing speed, memory, people skills, navigation, and intelligence. Lasting benefits have been documented up to 7 years later. Visit *www.BrainHQ.com*.

Environmental Relative Moldiness Index (ERMI)

The ERMI tests a sample of dust from your home or office for mold spores and provides a quantitative readout on dozens of mold species, as well as the likelihood that the level of mold found is problematic.

https://www.emlab.com/services/ermi-testing/ or
www.momsaware.org

Life Extension

A source for many online, "direct-to-consumer" lab tests at discount prices. Most tests are completed by LabCorp and results reported to you by LifeExtension. Further discounts are offered during their Annual Lab Test Sale, in April and May of each year.

www.lifeextension.com
Customer Service: 1-800-878-8989

International Society for Environmentally Acquired Illness

To find a physician trained in treating mold illness and other environmentally acquired illnesses, go to *https://iseai.org/find-a-professional/*.

Dr. Bredesen's Online "ReCODE Report"

A program of lab testing and personalized, computer print-out of recommendations.

https://www.ahnphealth.com/recode.html

Recommended Reading

Alter, Divya. *What to Eat for How You Feel: The New Kitchen — 100 Seasonal Recipes*. New York: Rizzoli, 2017.

Bredesen, D. *The End of Alzheimer's*. New York: Penguin Random House, 2017.

Guarneri, Mimi. *The Heart Speaks: A Cardiologist Reveals the Secret Language of Healing*. New York: Simon & Schuster, 2006.

Horner, Christine. *Radiant Health and Ageless Beauty: Dr. Christine Horner's 30-Day Program to Extraordinary Health, Beauty, and Longevity*. San Diego, CA: Elgea Publishing, 2016.

Hospodar, Miriam Kasin. *Heaven's Banquet: Vegetarian Cooking for Lifelong Health the Ayurveda Way*. New York: Penguin Random House, 2001.

Hyman, Mark. *The UltraMind Solution: Fix Your Broken Brain by Healing Your Body First*. New York: Simon & Schuster, 2008.

Lonsdorf, Nancy, Veronica Butler, and Melanie Brown. *A Woman's Best Medicine: Health, Happiness, and Long Life through Maharishi Ayur-Veda*. New York: Putman & Sons, revised, 1995.

Lonsdorf, Nancy. *The Ageless Woman; Natural Health and Beauty after Forty*. Fairfield, Iowa: Maharishi University of Management Press; second edition, 2016.

Mullin, Gerard E. The Gut Balance Revolution: Boost Your Metabolism, Restore Your Inner Ecology, and Lose the Weight for Good! Chicago, IL: Rodale Inc., 2015.

Perlmutter, David. *Grain Brain: The Surprising Truth about Wheat, Carbs, and Sugar — Your Brain's Silent Killers*. New York: Little, Brown & Company, 2013.

Pizzorno, Joseph. *The Toxin Solution: How Hidden Poisons in the Air, Water, Food, and Products We Use Are Destroying Our Health — AND WHAT WE CAN DO TO FIX IT*. New York: HarperOne, 2018.

Rosenthal, Norman E. *Transcendence: Healing and Transformation Through Transcendental Meditation*. New York: TarcherPerigree, 2012.

Roth, Bob. *Strength in Stillness: The Power of Transcendental Meditation*. New York: Simon & Schuster, 2018.

Steinbaum, Suzanne. *Dr. Suzanne Steinbaum's Heart Book: Every Woman's Guide to a Heart-Healthy Life*. New York: Avery, 2013.

Taubes, Gary. *The Case Against Sugar*. New York: Knopf, 2016.

Utian, Wulf. H. *Change your Menopause: Why One Size Does Not Fit All*. Beachwood, OH: Wulf H Utian LLC, 2011.

Wallace, Robert Keith and Samantha Wallace. *Gut Crisis: How Diet, Probiotics, and Friendly Bacteria Help You Lose Weight and Heal Your Body and Mind.* Fairfield, IA: Dharma Publications, 2017.

Yarema, T, et al. *Eat-Taste-Heal: An Ayurvedic Cookbook for Modern Living.* Kapaa, HI: Five Elements Press, 2006.

Yarema, Thomas, Daniel Rhoda, and Johnny Brannigan. *Eat-Taste-Heal: An Ayurvedic Cookbook for Modern Living.* 2006.

References

Chapter 1

Beason-Held, L. L., et al. Changes in Brain Function Occur Years before the Onset of Cognitive Impairment. *The Journal of Neuroscience*, 2013;*33*(46), 18008-18014. *http://doi.org/10.1523/JNEUROSCI.1402-13.2013.*

Bredesen, D. Reversal of cognitive decline: a novel therapeutic program. *Aging* 2014;Sep;6(9):707-17.

Bredesen, D. Metabolic profiling distinguishes three subtypes of Alzheimer's disease. *Aging* 2015; Aug;7(8):595-600.

Bredesen, D., et al., Reversal of cognitive decline in Alzheimer's disease. *Aging* 2016 Jun;8(6):1250-8. doi: 10.18632/aging.100981.

Bredesen, D., *The End of Alzheimer's*. Penguin Random House. New York, 2017.

Bredesen, D. and Rao, R. V. Ayurvedic Profiling of Alzheimer's Disease. *Altern Ther Health Med*. 2017 May;23(3):46-50. Epub 2017 Feb 27.

Crane, P., et al., Glucose Levels and Risk of Dementia. *New England Journal of Medicine*. 2013; Aug.8; 369(6): 540-548. doi: 10.1056/NEJMoa1215740.

DeKosky, S. and Gandy, S. Environmental Exposures and the Risk for Alzheimer Disease. *JAMA Neurol*. 2014 Mar; 71(3): 273-275. doi: 10.1001/jamaneurol.2013.6031.

DZNE - German Center for Neurodegenerative Diseases. Inflammation drives progression of Alzheimer's: A molecular complex of the immune system promotes aberrant aggregation of proteins. *ScienceDaily*. 2017 Dec. 20.

Gottesman, R.F., et al. Associations Between Midlife Vascular Risk Factors and 25-Year Incident Dementia in the Atherosclerosis Risk in Communities (ARIC) Cohort. *JAMA Neurol*. 2017 Aug 7. doi: 10.1001/jamaneurol.2017.1658.

Lipton, B. *The Wisdom of Your Cells: How Your Beliefs Control Your Biology*. Sounds True Publishing, Louisville, CO, 2006.

Lonsdorf, N. *The Ageless Woman*. Fairfield, Iowa: Maharishi University of Management Press; second edition, Fairfield, IA, 2016.

Morris, M.S. Homocysteine and Alzheimer's disease. *Lancet*. 2003 Jul;2(7):425-8.

Ramos-Cejudo, J. et al. Traumatic Brain Injury and Alzheimer's Disease: The Cerebrovascular Link. *EBioMedicine*. 2018 Feb; 28:21-30. doi: 10.1016/j.ebiom.2018.01.021.

Shaffer, J. Neuroplasticity and Clinical Practice: Building Brain Power for Health. *Front Psychol*. 2016; 7: 1118. doi: 10.3389/fpsyg.2016.01118.

Sharma, P. V. *Caraka Samhita*. 1981. Varanasi, India: Chaukahambha Orientalia.

Soscia, S. J., et. al. The Alzheimer's Disease-Associated Amyloid β-Protein Is an Antimicrobial Peptide. *Plos One,* 2010, *https://doi.org/10.1371/journal. pone.0009505.*

Venegas, C., et al. Microglia-derived ASC specks cross-seed amyloid-β in Alzheimer's disease. *Nature,* 2017; 552 (7685): 355 doi: 10.1038/nature25158.

Chapter 2

Abell, J., et al. Association between systolic blood pressure and dementia in the Whitehall II cohort study: role of age, duration, and threshold used to define hypertension. *European Heart Journal,* June 2018; https://doi. org/10.1093/eurheartj/ehy288.

Arnold, K., et al. Improving Diet Quality Is Associated with Decreased Inflammation: Findings from a Pilot Intervention in Postmenopausal Women with Obesity. *Journal of the Academy of Nutrition and Dietics* 2018;18 (ePublished).

Bai, Z., et al. Investigating the effect of transcendental meditation on blood pressure: a systematic review and meta-analysis. *J Hum Hypertens.* 2015 Nov;29(11):653-62. doi: 10.1038/jhh.2015.

Bisht, K., et al. Curcumin, resveratrol and flavonoids as anti-inflammatory, cyto- and DNA-protective dietary compounds. *Toxicology* 2010;278 (88-100).

Bowman, G. L., et al. Blood-brain barrier breakdown, neuroinflammation, and cognitive decline in older adults. *Alzheimer's & Dementia: the Journal of the Alzheimer's Association.* 2018;18 (3035-3038).

Flowers, E., et al. Prevalence of metabolic syndrome in South Asians residing in the United States. *Metabolic Syndrome and Related Disorders.* 2010; 8 (417-423).

Foulguier, S., et al. Hypertension-induced cognitive impairment: insights from prolonged angiotensin II infusion in mice. *Hypertension Research: Official Journal of the Japanese Society of Hypertension.* 2018; 10 (ePublished).

Gorelick, P. B., et al. Vascular contributions to cognitive impairment and dementia: a statement for healthcare professionals from the American Heart Association. *Stroke.* 2011; 42 (2672-2713).

Haring, B., et al. Cardiovascular disease and cognitive decline in postmenopausal women. *Journal of the American Heart Association.* 2013; 6: (e000369).

Kiran, U., et al. The role of Rajyoga meditation for modulation of anxiety and serum cortisol in patients undergoing coronary artery bypass surgery: A prospective randomized control study. *Annals of Cardiac Anesthesia.* 2017; 20 (158-162).

Lonsdorf, N. *The Ageless Woman*. Fairfield, Iowa: Maharishi University of Management Press; second edition, Fairfield, IA, 2016.

Maijo, M., et al. One-Year Consumption of a Mediterranean-Like Dietary Pattern With Vitamin D3 Supplements Induced Small Scale but Extensive Changes of Immune Cell Phenotype, Co-receptor Expression and Innate Immune Responses in Healthy Elderly Subjects: Results From the United Kingdom Arm of the NU-AGE Trial. *Frontiers in Physiology*. 2018; 997 (eCollection).

Norton, S., et al. Potential for primary prevention of Alzheimer's disease: an analysis of population-based data. *Lancet. 2014*; 8 (788-794).

Niwa Y. Effect of Maharishi 4 and Maharishi 5 on inflammatory mediators — with special reference to their free radical scavenging effect. *Indian J Clin Prac* 1991;1: 23-27.

Ornish, D. *Dr. Dean Ornish's Program for Reversing Heart Disease*. New York, NY: The Random House Publishing. 1996.

Ornish, D., et al. Can lifestyle changes reverse coronary heart disease? *Lancet*. 1990; 336 (129-133).

Ornish, D., et al. Changes in emerging cardiac biomarkers after an intensive lifestyle intervention. The American *Journal of Cardiology*. 2011; 108 (498-507).

Peter, L. Inflammation and cardiovascular disease mechanisms. *The American Journal of Clinical Nutrition*. 2006; 83 (456-460).

Piers, R. J. Structural brain volume differences between cognitively intact ApoE4 carriers and non-carriers across the lifespan. *Neural Regeneration Research*. 2018; 13 (1309-1312).

Rastogi, S., et al. Spices: Therapeutic Potential in Cardiovascular Health. *Current Pharmaceutical Design*. 2017; 23 (989-998).

Schneider, R., et al. A randomized controlled trial of stress reduction for hypertension in older African Americans. *Hypertension*. 1995; 26 (820-827).

Schneider, R., and Fields, J. *Total Heart Health: How to Prevent and Reverse Heart Disease with the Maharishi Vedic Approach to Health*. Laguna Beach, CA: Basic Health Publications. 2006.

Schrepf, A., et al. A multi-modal MRI study of the central response to inflammation in rheumatoid arthritis. *Nature Communications*. 2018; 9 (2243).

Sharma, H. M., et al. Inhibition of human low-density lipoprotein oxidation in vitro by Maharishi Ayur-Veda herbal mixtures. *Pharmacol Biochem Behav*. 1992 Dec;43(4):1175-82.

Shepherd-Banigan, M., et al. Improving vasomotor symptoms; psychological symptoms; and health-related quality of life in peri- or post-menopausal women through yoga: An umbrella systematic review and meta-analysis. *Complementary Therapies in Medicine*. 2017; 34 (156-164).

Shin, S., et al. Cognitive Impairment in Persons With Rheumatoid Arthritis. *Arthritis Care and Research*. 2013; 64 (1144-1150).

Siddharth, P., et al. Sedentary behavior associated with reduced medial temporal lobe thickness in middle-aged and older adults. *PLoS One*. 2018 Apr 12;13(4):e0195549. doi: 10.1371/journal.pone.0195549. eCollection 2018.

Smith, S. M., et al. Optimal Systolic Blood Pressure Target in Apparent Resistant and Non-Resistant Hypertension: A Pooled Analysis of Patient-Level Data from Sprint and ACCORD. *The American Journal of Medicine*. 2018;18 (ePublished).

Vohra, B. P., et al. Effect of Maharishi Amrit Kalash an ayurvedic herbal mixture on lipid peroxidation and neuronal lipofuscin accumulation in ageing guinea pig brain. *Indian J Exp Biol*. 2001 Apr;39(4):355-9.

Vohra, B. P., et al. Effect of Maharishi Amrit Kalash on age dependent variations in mitochondrial antioxidant enzymes, lipid peroxidation and mitochondrial population in different regions of the central nervous system of guinea-pigs. *Drug Metabol Drug Interact*. 2001;18(1):57-68.

Vohra, B. P., et al. Maharishi Amrit Kalash rejuvenates ageing central nervous system's antioxidant defense system: an in vivo study. *Pharmacol Res*. 1999 Dec; 40 (6): 497-502.

Wenyan, L., et al. Cerebrovascular Disease, Amyloid Plaques, and Dementia. *Stroke*. 2015;46:1402-1407. doi:10.1161/ STROKEAHA. 114.006571.

Chapter 3

Bala, S., et al. Acute binge drinking increases serum endotoxin and bacterial DNA levels in healthy individuals. *PLoS One*. 2014 May 14;9(5):e96864. doi: 10.1371/journal.pone.0096864. eCollection 2014.

Bonfili, L., et al. Microbiota modulation counteracts Alzheimer's disease progression influencing neuronal proteolysis and gut hormones plasma levels. *Scientific Reports*. 2017; 7 (24-26).

Campos, M., MD. *Leaky Gut: What is it, and what does it mean for you?* Harvard Health Publishing. 2017. Retrieved from *https://www.health.harvard.edu/blog/leaky-gut-what-is-it-and-what-does-it-mean-for-you-2017092212451*.

Drago, S., et al. Gliadin, zonulin and gut permeability: Effects on celiac and nonceliac intestinal mucosa and intestinal cell lines. *Scand J Gastroenterol*. 2006 Apr;41(4):40819.

Eke, B., et al. Effect of ingestion of microwaved foods on serum anti-oxidant enzymes and vitamins of albino rats. *Journal of Radiation Research and Applied Sciences*. Volume 10, Issue 2, April 2017, Pages 148-151. *https://doi. org/10.1016/j.jrras.2017.03.001*.

Editors of Encyclopedia Britannica. *The Vagus Nerve.* Encyclopedia Britannica. 2018. Retrieved from *https://www.britannica.com/science/vagus-nerve.*

Furness, J. *The Enteric Nervous System.* John Wiley & Sons. pp. 35-38. 2008.

Galland, L. The Gut Microbiome and the Brain. *Journal of Medicinal Food.* 2013; 17 (1261-1272).

Helena, S., et al. Oligodendrocyte, Astrocyte, and Microglia Crosstalk in Myelin Development, Damage, and Repair. *Frontiers in Cell and Developmental Biology.* 2016;28,June. doi:10.3389/fcell.2016.00071.

Kho, Z., and Lal, S. The Human Gut Microbiome – A Potential Controller of Wellness and Disease. *Frontiers in Microbiology.* 2018; August 2018 I Volume 9 I Article 1835.

Kunnumakkara, A. B., et al. Chronic diseases, inflammation, and spices: how are they linked? *Journal of Translational Medicine.* 2018; 16 (14-39).

Luan, H. et al. Mass spectrometry-based metabolomics: Targeting the crosstalk between gut microbiota and brain in neurodegenerative disorders. *Mass Spectrom Rev.* 2017 Nov 12. doi: 10.1002/mas.21553.

McCabe, L., et al. Prebiotic and Probiotic Regulation of Bone Health: Role of the Intestine and its Microbiome. *Curr Osteoporos.* 2015; Rep 13 (363-371).

McFarli, B., et al. Oral spore-based probiotic supplementation was associated with reduced incidence of post-prandial dietary endotoxin, triglycerides, and disease risk biomarkers. *World J Gastrointest Pathophysiol.* 2017 August 15; 8(3): 117-126.

Patel, H., et al. Structural and enzyme kinetic studies of retrograded starch: Inhibition of α-amylase and consequences for intestinal digestion of starch. *Elsevier Journal.* 2017; 164 (154-161).

Rao, R. V., et al. Ayurvedic medicinal plants for Alzheimer's disease: a review. *Alzheimer's Research & Therapy* 2012, 4:22. http://alzres.com/content/4/3/22.

Raj, D., et al. Increased White Matter Inflammation in Aging- and Alzheimer's Disease Brain. *Frontiers in Molecular Neuroscience.* 2017; 10 (Article 206).

Sampson, T., and Mazmanian, S. Control of Brain Development, Function, and Behavior by the Microbiome. *Cell Host & Microbe.* 2015;17 (565-576).

Severance, E. G., et al. Gastroenterology issues in schizophrenia: why the gut matters. *Current Psychology.* 2015; Rep 17 (25-41).

Sonnenburg, J., and Sonnenburg, E. *The Good Gut: Taking Control of Your Weight, Your Mood, and Your Long-term Health.* Penguin Books. 2015.

Sturgeon, C., et al. Zonulin transgenic mice show altered gut permeability and increased morbidity/mortality in the DSS colitis model. *Ann N Y Acad Sci.* 2017 June; 1397(1): 130-142. doi:10.1111/nyas.13343.

Tiwari, P., et al. Recapitulation of Ayurveda constitution types by machine learning of phenotypic traits. *PLoS One.* 2017 Oct 5;12(10):e0185380. doi: 10.1371/journal.pone.0185380. eCollection 2017.

Vogt, N. et al. Gut microbiome alterations in Alzheimer's disease. *Scientific Reports*. 2017; October 19. doi:10.1038/s41598-017-13601-y.

Westfall., S., et al. Longevity extension in Drosophila through gut-brain communication. *Scientific Reports*. 2018; 8 (47-62).

Yano, J. M., et al. Indigenous Bacteria from the Gut Microbiota Regulate Host Serotonin Biosynthesis. *Cell Press*. 2015; 161 (264-276).

Chapter 4

Abildgaard, J., et al. Ectopic lipid deposition is associated with insulin resistance in postmenopausal women. *The Journal of Clinical Endocrinology and Metabolism*. 2018; 10 (1210-1225).

Beam, C. R., et al. Differences Between Women and Men in Incidence Rates of Dementia and Alzheimer's Disease. *Journal of Alzheimer's Disease*. 2018; 64 (1077-1083).

Bhanpuri, N. H., et al. Cardiovascular disease risk factor responses to a type 2 diabetes care model including nutritional ketosis induced by sustained carbohydrate restriction at 1 year: an open label, non-randomized, controlled study. *Cardiovascular Diabetology*. 2018;17 (1-16).

Boland, B., et al. Promoting the clearance of neurotoxic proteins in neurodegenerative disorders of ageing. *Nature Reviews Drug Discovery*. 2018;109 (10-17).

Bowman, G. L., et al. Blood-brain barrier breakdown, neuroinflammation, and cognitive decline in older adults. *Alzheimer's & Dementia: The Journal of the Alzheimer's Association*. 2018; 18 (3035-3038).

Bredesen, B. *ReCode Report* Accessed at *https://www.drbredesen.com/participants*. 2017.

Congdon, E. Sex Differences in Autophagy Contribute to Female Vulnerability in Alzheimer's Disease. *Frontiers in Neuroscience*. 2018; 12 (372-380).

De La Monte, S. Brain insulin resistance and deficiency as therapeutic targets in Alzheimer's disease. *Curr Alzheimer Res*. 2012 Jan;9(1):35-66.

De La Monte, S. Brain metabolic dysfunction at the core of Alzheimer's disease. *Biochem Pharmacol*. 2014 Apr 15;88(4):548-59. doi: 10.1016/j.bcp.2013.12.012. Epub 2013 Dec 28.

De La Monte, S. Contributions of brain insulin resistance and deficiency in amyloid-related neurodegeneration in Alzheimer's disease. *Drugs*. 2012 Jan 1;72(1):49-66. doi: 10.2165/11597760-000000000-00000.

De La Monte, S. Epidemiological trends strongly suggest exposures as etiologic agents in the pathogenesis of sporadic Alzheimer's disease, diabetes mellitus, and non-alcoholic steatohepatitis. *J Alzheimers Dis*. 2009;17(3):519-29. doi: 10.3233/JAD-2009-1070.

Dong, S., et al. Berberine Could Ameliorate Cardiac Dysfunction via Interfering Myocardial Lipidomic Profiles in the Rat Model of Diabetic Cardiomyopathy. *Frontiers in Physiology.* 2018 (e-collection).

Eissa, L. A., et al. Antioxidant and anti-inflammatory activities of berberine attenuate hepatic fibrosis induced by thioacetamide injection in rats. *Journal of Chemico-biological Interactions* (e-pub). 2018.

Ezquerro, S., et al. Ghrelin reduces TNF-α-induced human hepatocyte apoptosis, autophagy and pyroptosis: role in obesity-associated NAFLD. *Journal of Clinical Endocrine Metabolism*; 2018; 10 (171-182).

Fink, R. I., et al. Mechanisms of Insulin Resistance in Aging. *Journal of Clinical Investigation.* 1983; 71 (1523-1535).

Gao, Y., et al. FOXO3 Inhibits Human Gastric Adenocarcinoma (AGS) Cell Growth by Promoting Autophagy in an Acidic Microenvironment. *Cell Physiology Biochemistry.* 2018; 49 (335-348).

Ge, Q., et al. Treatment of Diabetes Mellitus Using iPS Cells and Spice Polyphenols. *Journal of Diabetes Research* 2017 (1-11).

Goyal, S. K., et al. Stevia (Stevia rebaudiana) a bio-sweetener: a review. *Int J Food Sci Nutr.* 2010 Feb;61(1):1-10. doi: 10.3109/09637480903193049.

Guilliams, T. *Supplementing Dietary Nutrients A Guide for Healthcare Professionals.* Point Institute. 2017.

Harrar, S. Insulin Resistance Causes and Symptoms. Accessed at *https://www.endocrineweb.com/conditions/type-2-diabetes/insulin-resistance-causes-symptoms.* 2016.

Kassaar, O., et al. Macrophage Migration Inhibitory Factor is subjected to glucose modification and oxidation in Alzheimer's Disease. *Scientific Reports.* 2017; 7 (1-11).

Kearns, C. E., et al. Sugar Industry and Coronary Heart Disease Research: A Historical Analysis of Internal Industry Documents. *JAMA Intern Med.*2016; 176 (1680-1685).

Lange, K. W., et al. Ketogenic diets and Alzheimer's Disease. *Food Science and Human Wellness. 2016;* 6 (1-9).

Levy, A., et al. Co-sensitivity to the incentive properties of palatable food and cocaine in rats; implications for co-morbid addictions. *Addiction Biology.* 2013. 18 (763-773).

Lonsdorf, N. *The Ageless Woman.* Fairfield, Iowa: Maharishi University of Management Press; second edition, Fairfield, IA, 2016.

Ma, Y., et al. Expression of autophagy-related genes in cerebrospinal fluid of patients with tuberculous meningitis. *Experimental and Therapeutic Medicine.* 2018; 15 (4671-4676).

Minta, W., et al. Estrogen deprivation aggravates cardiometabolic dysfunction in obese-insulin resistant rats through the impairment of cardiac mitochondrial dynamics. *Experimental Gerontology*. 2018; 103 (107-114).

Monte, S., and Wands, J. Alzheimer's Disease Is Type 3 Diabetes—Evidence Reviewed. *Journal of Diabetes Science and Technology*; 2008; 6 (1101-1113).

Oboh, G., et al. Inhibitory Effect of Garlic, Purple Onion, and White Onion on Key Enzymes Linked with Type 2 Diabetes and Hypertension. *Journal of Dietary Supplements*. 2018; 9 (1-14).

Pae, M., et al. Loss of ovarian function in association with a high-fat diet promotes insulin resistance and disturbs adipose tissue immune homeostasis. *The Journal of Nutritional Biochemistry*. 2018; 57 (93-102).

Pradeep, S. R., and Srinivasan, K. Ameliorative Influence of Dietary Fenugreek (Trigonella foenum-graecum) Seeds and Onion (Allium cepa) on Eye Lens Abnormalities via Modulation of Crystallin Proteins and Polyol Pathway in Experimental Diabetes. *Current Eye Research*. 2018; 43 (1108-1118).

Sakkiah, S., et al. Endocrine Disrupting Chemicals Mediated through Binding Androgen Receptor Are Associated with Diabetes Mellitus. *Int J Environ Res Public Health*. 2017 Dec 23;15(1). pii: E25. doi: 10.3390/ijerph15010025.

Shin, B. K., et al. Intermittent fasting protects against the deterioration of cognitive function, energy metabolism and dyslipidemia in Alzheimer's disease-induced estrogen deficient rats. *Journal of Experimental Biology and Medicine*. 2018; 243 (334-343).

Singh, D. K., et al. Hypolipidaemic Effects of Gymnema sylvestre on High Fat Diet Induced Dyslipidaemia in Wistar Rats. *Journal of Clinical and Diagnostic Research*. 2017; 5 (FF01-FF05).

Zhang, Z., et al. Inhibition of glycogen synthase kinase-3β by Angelica sinensis extract decreases β-amyloid-induced neurotoxicity and tau phosphorylation in cultured cortical neurons. *J Neurosci Res*. 2011 Mar;89(3):437-47. doi: 10.1002/jnr.22563. Epub 2010 Dec 17.

Zeevi, D., et al. Personalized Nutrition by Prediction of Glycemic Responses. *Cell*. 2015 Nov 19;163(5):1079-1094. doi: 10.1016/j.cell.2015.11.001.

Chapter 5

Bito, T., et. al. Characterization and Quantitation of Vitamin B12 Compounds in Various Chlorella Supplements. *Journal of Agricultural and Food Chemistry*, 2016; 64(45):8516-8524. Epub 2016 Nov 2.

Bjelland, I., et al. Lowering blood homocysteine with folic acid-based supplements: meta-analysis of randomized trials. *Archives of General Psychiatry*. 2003;60(6):618-626. doi:10.1001/archpsyc.60.6.618

Bredesen, D., *The End of Alzheimer's*. 2017. Penguin Random House, NY.

Brewer, G. J. Copper excess, zinc deficiency, and cognition loss in Alzheimer's disease. *Biofactors 2012. 38*:107-113, doi:10.1002/biof.1005.

Cacabelos, R., et al. Therapeutic effects of Citicoline in Alzheimer's disease. Cognition, brain mapping, cerebrovascular hemodynamics, and immune factors. *Annals of the New York Academy of Sciences. 1996*; 777, 399-403.

Douaud, G., et al. Preventing Alzheimer's disease-related gray matter atrophy by B-vitamin treatment. *Proceedings of the National Academy of Sciences of the United States of America.* 2013; Jun4; 110(23): 9523-9528.

Dyall, C. S. Long-chain omega-3 fatty acids and the brain: a review of the independent and shared effects of EPA, DPA and DHA. *Front Aging Neurosci. 2015;7:52.*

Hanna, S., et al. Vitamin B12 Deficiency and Depression in the Elderly: Review and Case Report. *Primary Care Companion to The Journal of Clinical Psychiatry.* 2009; 11(5), 269-270. doi:10.4088/PCC.08100707.

Gangwisch, J. E., et al. National Longitudinal Study of Adolescent Health, USA, 1994-1996; *Sleep,* Vol. 33, No. 1, 2010.

Gareri, P., and Castagna, A. Citicoline as Add-On Treatment in Alzheimer's Disease: Tips from the Citicholinage Study. *J Alzheimers Dis Parkinsonism* 2017, 7:4 doi: 10.4172/2161-0460.1000353.

Li, W., et al. Elevation of brain magnesium prevents synaptic loss and reverses cognitive deficits in Alzheimer's disease mouse model. *Molecular Brain.* 2014;7:65. doi:10.1186/s13041-014-0065-y.

Long, E., et al. Homocysteine Lowering with Folic Acid and B Vitamins in Vascular Disease. *New England Journal of Medicine*; 2006; 354:1567-1577. doi: 10.1056/NEJMoa06090.

Mercola, J. *Effortless Healing, 9 Simple Ways to Sidestep Illness, Shed Excess Weight and Help Your Body Fix Itself.* 2015. Hay House UK Ltd. London, England.

Narayan, P., et al. Effects of pulsating magnetic fields on the physiology of animals and man. *Current Science.* 1984;53 (18): 959-965.

Rao, R. V., Descamps, O., John, V., and Bredesen, D. E. Ayurvedic medicinal plants for Alzheimer's disease: a review. *Alzheimer's Research & Therapy*; 2012; 4(3), 22. http://doi.org/10.1186/alzrt125.

Reynolds, E. H. Folic acid, ageing, depression, and dementia. *BMJ: British Medical Journal.* 2002; 324(7352):1512-1515.

Smith, D., et. al. Homocysteine-Lowering by B Vitamins Slows the Rate of Accelerated Brain Atrophy in Mild Cognitive Impairment: A Randomized Controlled Trial. *PLoS One.* 2010;5(9):e12244. doi: 10.1371/journal.pone.0012244.

Smorgon, C., et al. Trace elements and cognitive impairment: an elderly cohort study. *Archives of Gerontology and Geriatric Supplement 9;* 2004;393-402. doi: 10.1016/j.archger.2004.04.050.

Romm, A., et al. *Botanical Medicine for Women's Health.* 2010. Elsevier Inc. St. Louis, MO. *https://doi.org/10.1016/B978-0-443-07277-2.X0001-3.*

Tucker, K., Are you vitamin B12 deficient? *Agricultural Research magazine.* August 2000.

Wurtman, R. J. A nutrient combination that can affect synapse formation. *Nutrients.* 2014 Apr 23;6(4):1701-10. doi: 10.3390/nu6041701.

Yang, F., et al. Curcumin inhibits formation of amyloid beta oligomers and fibrils, binds plaques, and reduces amyloid in vivo. *J Biol Chem.* 2005 Feb 18;280(7):5892-901. Epub 2004 Dec 7.PMID: 15590663.

Chapter 6

Alirezaei, M., et al. Short-term fasting induces profound neuronal autophagy. *Autophagy.* 2010;6(6):702-710. doi:10.4161/auto.6.6.12376.

Asarnow, L. D., et al. The Effects of Bedtime and Sleep Duration on Academic and Emotional Outcomes in a Nationally Representative Sample of Adolescents, *Journal of Adolescent Health,* Volume 54, Issue 3, 350-356.

Bodel, P., et al. Anti-inflammatory effects of estradiol on human blood leukocytes. *J Lab and Clin Medicine.* 1972 Sept. Vol 80, No 3, pp 373-384.

Bossy, B., et al. Clearing the Brain's Cobwebs: The Role of Autophagy in Neuroprotection. *Current Neuropharmacology.* 2008; 6(2): 97-101. doi: 10.2174/157015908784533897.

Chrousos, G. P., Stress and disorders of the stress system. *Nature Reviews Endocrinology.* 2009; 5(7), 374-381. doi: 10.1038/nrendo.2009.106.

Coetsee, C., and Terblanche, E. The effect of three different exercise training modalities on cognitive and physical function in a healthy older population. *European Review of Aging and Physical Activity.* 2017;14:13. doi:10.1186/s11556-017-0183-5.

Deichmann, R., et al. Coenzyme Q10 and Statin-Induced Mitochondrial Dysfunction. *The Ochsner Journal.* 2010;10(1):16-21.

Du, J. Y., et al. Percutaneous Progesterone Delivery Via Cream or Gel Application in Postmenopausal Women, A Randomized, Crossover Study of Progesterone Levels in Serum, Whole Blood, Saliva and Capillary Blood. *Menopause,* 2013;20(11):1169-1175.

Duvivier, B. M. F. M., et al. Reducing sitting time versus adding exercise: differential effects on biomarkers of endothelial dysfunction and metabolic risk. *SCI Rep.* 2018 Jun 5;8(1):8657. doi: 10.1038/s41598-018-26616-w.

Edwards, J., et al. Cognitive training and selective attention in the aging brain: An electrophysiological study. *Clinical Neurophysiology.* November 2013; volume 124,issue11: 2198-2208. *https://doi.org/10.1016/j.clinph.2013.05.012. https://www.sciencedirect.com/science/article/pii/B012227055X007665.*

Ford, F. Premenstrual syndrome: nutritional aspects. *Encyclopedia of Food Sciences and Nutrition.* 2003 (Second Edition).

Garaulet, M., et al. Timing of food intake predicts weight loss effectiveness. *International Journal of Obesity.* April 2013; 37, 604-611.

Gomes-Osman, J., et al. Exercise for cognitive brain health in aging: A systematic review for an evaluation of dose. *Neurology: Clinical Practice.* 2018; 8. 257-265. 10.1212/CPJ.0000000000000460.

Greendale, G. A., et al. Effects of the menopause transition and hormone use on cognitive performance in midlife women. *Neurology.* 2009;72(21):1850-1857.

KEEPS Report. Presented at 2012 North American Menopause Society Annual Meeting. October 3-6. Orlando FL.

Lonsdorf, N. *The Ageless Woman.* Fairfield, Iowa: Maharishi University of Management Press; second edition, Fairfield, IA, 2016.

Maki, P. Is Timing Everything? New Insights into Why the Effect of Estrogen Therapy on Memory Might be Age Dependent. *Endocrinology.* 2013. 154(8), 2570-2572. *http://doi.org/10.1210/en.2013-1598.*

Manson, J. E., et al. Menopausal Hormone Therapy and Health Outcomes During the Intervention and Extended Poststopping Phases of the Women's Health Initiative Randomized Trials. *JAMA.* 2013 Oct 2;310(13):1353-68. doi: 10.1001/jama.2013.278040.

McArthur, J. O., et al. Biological variability and impact of oral contraceptives on vitamins B(6), B(12) and folate status in women of reproductive age. *Nutrients.* 2013 Sep 16;5(9):3634-45. doi: 10.3390/nu50936.

McEwen, B. S., and Lasley, E. N. *The end of stress as we know it.* 2002. Washington, D.C: Joseph Henry Press.

Mikkola, T. S. New evidence for cardiac benefit of postmenopausal hormone therapy. *Climacteric.* 2017 Feb;20(1):5-10.

Mikkola, T. S., et al. Estradiol-based postmenopausal hormone therapy and risk of cardiovascular and all-cause mortality. *Menopause.* 2015, Vol. 22, No. 9, pp. 976-983.

Mosconi, L., et al. Sex differences in Alzheimer risk: Brain imaging of endocrine vs chronologic aging. *Neurology.* 2017; Sep 26;89(13):1382-1390. doi: 10.1212/WNL.0000000000004425. Epub 2017 Aug 30.

Orme-Johnson D. W., and Walton, K. G. All approaches to preventing or reversing effect of stress are not the same. *American Journal of Health Promotion.* 1998;12: 297-299.

Osterberg, K. L., et al. Effect of acute resistance exercise on post-exercise oxygen consumption and resting metabolic rate in young women. *Int J Sport Nutr Exerc Metab. https://www.ncbi.nlm.nih.gov/pubmed/10939877* 2000 Mar;10(1):71-81.

Palmery, M., et al. Oral contraceptives and changes in nutritional requirements. *Eur Rev Med Pharmacol Sci.* 2013 Jul;17(13):1804-13.

Ratey, J. *Spark, The Revolutionary New Science of Exercise and the Brain.* 2008. Gildan Media Corp Boston, MA.

Rosenthal, N. E., *Transcendence: Healing and Transformation through Transcendental Meditation,* 2012, Tarcher/Putnam, New York.

Scullin, M. K., and Bliwise, D. L. Sleep, cognition, and normal aging: integrating a half century of multidisciplinary research. *Perspect Psychol Sci.* 2015 Jan;10(1):97-137. doi: 10.1177/1745691614556680.

Sharma, P.V. *Caraka Samhit.* 1981. Varanasi, India: Chaukahambha Orientalia.

Silverman, D.H., et al. Differences in Regional Brain Metabolism Associated with Specific Formulations of Hormone Therapy in Postmenopausal Women at Risk for AD. *Psychoneuroendocrinology.* 2011 May; 36(4): 502-513.

Sleiman, S. F., et al. Exercise promotes the expression of brain derived neurotrophic factor (BDNF) through the action of the ketone body β-hydroxybutyrate. Elmquist JK, ed. *eLife.* 2016;5:e15092. doi:10.7554/eLife.15092.

Stephanick, M., et al. The Women's Health Initiative Postmenopausal Hormone Trials: Overview and Baseline Characteristics of Participants, *Ann Epidemiol* 2003;13:S78-S86.

Tannen, R. L., et al. Perspectives on Hormone Replacement Therapy: The Women's Health Initiative and New Observational Studies Sampling the Overall Population. *Fertil Steril.* 2008 August; 90(2): 258-264.

Travis, F., and Arenander, A. Cross-sectional and longitudinal study of effects of transcendental meditation practice on interhemispheric frontal asymmetry and frontal coherence. *International Journal of Neuroscience.* 2006;116(12):1519-38. PMID:17145686. doi:10.1080/00207450600575482 .*https://doi.org/10.1080/00207450600575482*

Vernikos, J. *Sitting Kills, Moving Heals: How Simple Everyday Movement Will Prevent Pain, Illness, and Early Death.* 2011. Quill Driver Books. Fresno, CA.

Wharton, W., et al. Potential role of estrogen in the pathobiology and prevention of Alzheimer's disease. American *Journal of Translational Research.* 2009;1(2):131-137.

William, J., et al. Cognitive Behavioral Treatment of Insomnia. *Chest.* 2013 Feb; 143(2): 554-565. doi: 10.1378/chest.12-0731.

Wolinsky, F. D., et al. A randomized controlled trial of cognitive training using a visual speed of processing intervention in middle aged and older adults. *PLoS One.* 2013, May 1;8(5):e61624. doi: 10.1371/journal. pone.0061624.

Xie, L., et al. Sleep initiated fluid flux drives metabolite clearance from the adult brain. *Science,* October 18, 2013. doi: 10.1126/science.1241224.

Yaffe, C., et al. Connection between sleep and cognition in older adults. *Lancet.* 2014; volume 13, issue 10 p. 1017-1028. *https://doi.org/10.1016/ S1474-4422(14)70172-3.*

Chapter 7

Balstad, T. R., et al. Coffee, broccoli and spices are strong inducers of electrophile. *Mol Nutr Food Res.* 2011 Feb;55(2):185-97. doi: 10.1002/ mnfr.201000204. Epub 2010 Sep 8.

Bredesen, D. E. Inhalational Alzheimer's disease: an unrecognized—and treatable—epidemic. *Aging* (Albany NY). 2016;8(2):304-313.

Cacciottolo, M., et al. Particulate air pollutants, APOE alleles and their contributions to cognitive impairment in older women and to amyloidogenesis in experimental models. *Translational Psychiatry.* 2017; 7. e1022. 10.1038/ tp.2016.280.

Calderón-Garcidueñas L., et al. Prefrontal white matter pathology in air pollution exposed Mexico City young urbanites and their potential impact on neurovascular unit dysfunction and the development of Alzheimer's disease. *International Journal of Environmental Research and Public Health.* 2016; Apr;146:404-17.

Conzade, R., et al., Prevalence and Predictors of Subclinical Micronutrient Deficiency in German Older Adults: Results from the Population-Based KORA-Age Study. *Nutrients.* 2017: Dec; 9(12): 1276. doi: 10.3390/ nu9121276.

Goldinger, A., et al. Seasonal Effects on Gene Expression. *PLoS ONE.* 2015; 10(5): e0126995. doi:10.1371/journal.pone.0126995.

Herron, R. E., and Fagan, J. B. Lipophil-mediated reduction of toxicants in humans: an evaluation of an ayurvedic detoxification procedure. *Altern Ther Health Med.* 2002 Sep-Oct;8(5):40-51. PMID:12233802.

Hodges, R. E., and Minich, D. M. Modulation of Metabolic Detoxification Pathways Using Foods and Food-Derived Components: A Scientific Review with Clinical Application, *Journal of Nutrition and Metabolism,* vol. 2015, Article ID 760689, 23 pages, 2015. doi:10.1155/2015/760689.

Kubsad, D., et al. Assessment of Glyphosate Induced Epigenetic Transgenerational Inheritance of Pathologies and Sperm Epimutations: Generational Toxicology. *Scientific Reports,* 2019. 9. 10.1038/s41598-019-42860-0.

Lorenz, I., et al. Increased plasma levels of matrix metalloproteinase-9 in patients with Alzheimer's disease. *Neurochem Int.* 2003 Aug;43(3):191-6. PMID: 12689599.

Luckenbach, T., et al. Fatal attraction: synthetic musk fragrances compromise multixenobiotic defense systems in mussels. *Mar Environ Res.* 2004 Aug-Dec;58(2-5):215-9.

Oulhaj, A., et al., Omega-3 Fatty Acid Status Enhances the Prevention of Cognitive Decline by B Vitamins in Mild Cognitive Impairment. *Journal of Alzheimer's Disease.* 2016; 50(2): 547-557. doi: 10.3233/JAD-150777. PMID: 26757190.

Rao, R. V., et al. Ayurvedic medicinal plants for Alzheimer's disease: a review. *Alzheimer's Research & Therapy;* 2012, 4:22. *http://alzres.com/content/4/3/22.*

Hodges, R. E., and Minich, D. M. Modulation of Metabolic Detoxification Pathways Using Foods and Food-Derived Components: A Scientific Review with Clinical Application, *Journal of Nutrition and Metabolism*, vol. 2015, Article ID 760689, 23 pages, 2015. doi:10.1155/2015/760689.

US Environmental Protection Agency, Research and Development. Toxic Trace Metals in Human and Mammalian Hair and Nails. *EPA-600.* 1979;4.79-049, August 1979.

Xaquin, C., et al. Widespread seasonal gene expression reveals annual differences in human immunity and physiology. *Nature Communications* 6, Article number: 7000 (2015), doi:10.1038/ncomms8000.

About the Author

Nancy Lonsdorf, MD, is a Johns Hopkins- and Stanford-trained physician who has pioneered an integrative medical approach using Ayurveda, functional medicine and Western medicine over the past 30 years. Specializing in women's health, she is the co-author of *A Woman's Best Medicine,* a handbook of Ayurvedic wisdom for women of all ages, and author of *The Ageless Woman*, a woman's guide to navigating menopause smoothly, using Ayurveda and natural approaches.

In addition to her dedicated patient work, Dr. Lonsdorf has appeared frequently on national television and radio and contributes to many popular publications, including *Natural Solutions, Yoga International, Yoga Journal,* and *First for Women.* She is a sought-after international speaker, teaches Integrative Medicine and Maharishi Ayurveda to health professionals, and is a compelling online physician-educator dedicated to empowering women with the knowledge and support they need to restore and maintain vibrant health from within.

Dr. Lonsdorf is certified as a Bredesen ReCODE practitioner and now focuses her work on preventing and reversing cognitive decline naturally, and on making Alzheimer's disease just a memory.

Made in the USA
Coppell, TX
02 December 2019

12276822R00178